A Way Out
Of Pain
And Stress

The Healing Effects
Of
Craniosacral Therapy

By: Annette Eccles, LMT

This book is dedicated to my clients who have shared their personal journeys with me and inspired me to trust the human body, intuition and a higher power than myself that guides my work. Some of these paths have been relatively simple and straight forward, others difficult and complicated. But all have humbled me. For that I thank each of you.

Table of Contents

Introduction

An Invitation To Healing

Do you remember those carefree days as a child when your greatest concern was the decision whether you would ride your bike or go swimming? Remember when it didn't matter if your shorts came from a department store? They didn't have a certain label printed on the outside and your bike didn't have to be an Audi or a Benz. When laughter came easily and there was nothing more inviting than the soft blue sky, the warmth of the shining sun and the promise of another day's adventure.

And now... if you're like most adults, stress is rampant, tension is high and living with pain or taking prescription drugs seems to be the norm.

So when did things change? Was it in high school when you were trying so hard to get the lead role in that theatrical production, or maybe trying to make first string on the football field so you could feel the thrill of those Friday night lights, the cheer of the crowd and the girls' admiring eye? Perhaps you awakened one morning with college midterms looming ahead of you and realizing your stomach felt tied in knots while your dinner from the previous night feeling like it was nails mixed in dirty grey sludge. Or was it when you finally got that coveted job and realized the expectations were through the roof. That night you went home from work with a killer headache that felt like someone was driving a wooden stake right through your temple.

Like so many people, you probably can't put a finger on when life became challenging-- but now you are on Lipitor for high blood pressure, and Xanex for the acid burning up your stomach, oh and don't forget to pick up the Imitrex prescription in case your migraines decide to spend the night with you again.

Somehow you suspect that SOMETHING ELSE is at the core of your problems…or maybe you're not thrilled with being on medications. But – what else can you do?

I've been involved in the field of dentistry for the past 20 years. I started as a registered dental assistant, and worked in every aspect of a dental office as well as consulting in many offices. However, the more I learned about dentistry and health in general, I realized there is more to achieving a healthy body than healing symptoms and chasing pain. I wanted to learn more and to understand why it seemed that symptoms often times originate from somewhere totally different than indicated by malfunction or pain. I was put in contact with the Upledger Institute in Palm Beach, Florida and it was love at first touch. I soon discovered that as a craniosacral therapist I would be acting as more of a facilitator than a practitioner. What I mean by this concept is that almost all other practitioners whether it be a doctor, a

2

chiropractor, a physical therapist or a massage therapist attempts to figure out what is wrong with the body and then manipulate that body by either manual manipulation or the use of drugs or herbs, trying to tell the body what to do to get better. Whereas a craniosacral therapist simply tries to create and hold an environment where the body can heal itself, trusting it has the innate ability to do so. This is done by quietly listening to what the body tells the therapist through touch. This may not make much sense to you now but I will get into great depth on this subject later in the book. I admired and believed in this philosophy so I completed a degree in medical massage with a focus on craniosacral therapy, as well as certifications in both somato emotional release and lymphatic drainage therapy. Because movement is such an important part of a healthy body, I also became certified for teaching Pilates Mat and Reformer from Polestar Neuromuscular Education System.

In this book we will look at new and proven ways of improving your health and finding options to your medical issues. In actuality the concepts we will discuss are not new but have been rediscovered in the recent past. These concepts include systems of the body that affect your overall health and well-being. So if you are new to the world of alternative medicine this book will give you an in depth over view of evidences and case studies to show its validity as well as how it can help you feel better and live a more abundant life style. Or perhaps you have dipped your toe into the pond of alternative medicine but not found quite the comfort or success you were hoping to achieve. Then this information will deepen your understanding and explain why there are certain steps a person must take to achieve the most optimal results.

Jane was a 55 year old female who suffered from depression to the point of not being able to complete normal every day activities due to overwhelming feelings of listlessness, hopelessness and fatigue.

Ricky was a seven year old boy who had speech problems, developing symptoms of ADD and being labeled as a problem student.

Steve was a 33 year old active male who enjoyed doing triathlons until three years previous when his body began to break down. Now his body seemed to be one cramp or another or enough pain to keep him from his beloved past time.

Aaron was a 53 year old retired Army special operations leader who now suffered with chronic pain, insomnia, and mild post-traumatic stress syndrome. He felt as though he couldn't turn off his brain anymore even though his current career was not of a stressful nature.

Perhaps you can relate to David, Jane or Ricky's situation or maybe at your last doctor's visit you experienced this familiar situation. You tried to tell your doctor things just weren't feeling right in your body and that you're always tired. He asked if you were feeling any pain and if so where. "All over, but mostly just not feeling right," was your reply. He did a quick cursory exam and reported all seemed fine. He then ordered routine blood work and recommended you decrease the stress in your life. Yes, you are all for that, but really, what are you going to cut out? Work?! Then to your relief and discouragement the test results came back and were all "within the normal limits". When your doctor called to give you the good news that nothing was wrong you protested asking, "Then why don't I feel right?" His response surprised you and frustrated you, "Would you like to try an anti-depressant? It will help you sleep better and even cope better with your daily stress. Perhaps if we do that for a short period of time you will feel better." You feel as though, yes that might help you feel better but does it really tell you what is wrong with you? And what if it helps resolve one issue but creates other issues?

Many people in the United States are finding this to be a typical scenario when they visit their physicians. So often there isn't an answer that addresses the root of your health care issues but seems to be an educated guessing game of which medication will get rid of what symptom. This only gives rise to the question of "will this new medicine interact with other medications that a different specialist has put me on, creating even more symptoms?"

Imagine if you will that you receive an overdraft notice from your bank. When you look at it you're shocked because you know you have plenty of money in your checking account. Understanding dawns when you review a transaction report with the bank supervisor. Your daughter who is attending college, out of state, has used her emergency debit card to purchase something. The bank supervisor understands the situation and the fact that you have been a loyal client, so she deletes the overdraft charges on your account. You transfer money from savings into checking and all is resolved.....until two weeks later when you receive yet another overdraft notice. Again you go to the bank only to find the same problem has arisen. At this point, do you just keep transferring money from savings to checking and paying overdraft charges or do you have a heartfelt discussion with your daughter on the meaning of "emergency" and tell her she has to have the emergency approved by you before using her debit card so that you can make sure the checking account can handle the deduction? In other words do you take care of the issue that is causing the problem or do you just keep dealing with the symptom of being over-drawn? I venture to say you would deal with the underlying issue causing the problem. If not, can I have an emergency debit card from your checking account?

Back to your office visit with your physician, at what point do you ask yourself the difficult questions, "Does this system make sense for me?" "Am I getting to the core issues of my health concerns?" "Where are these visits and medications leading to?" "Is this what I want my life to be like?" "Is this all there is to my life?"

What Western Medicine Does and Doesn't Do

Allopathic medicine, the traditional medical system most of us are familiar with is a system of medical practices that aim to combat disease by use of remedies such as drugs or surgery, producing effects different from or incompatible with those produced by the disease (medical definition by dictitionary.com). With all of the discoveries over the years this type of medical care does an amazing job with emergency medicine and especially trauma medicine. All you have to do is see a person mutilated in an automobile accident and watch what an excellently trained trauma surgeon does to put them back together again to appreciate the knowledge and skills modern medicine provides for us. Or if you have ever had a loved one suffer a heart attack, have paramedics use equipment to restore their heart beat to maintain life, and then have a cardiac surgeon repair the heart and stabilize this loved one, you will express gratitude for the machines, training, medications and response systems we enjoy as part of our culture today. The advancements in technology and surgery are incredible.

I want to make it clear here that I am not anti-medical. I even have a son and several friends who are medical doctors. I admire them for their dedication and sacrifice over the years to get through medical school and then try to work within a broken system to try to help individuals feel better. Even though I rarely use an allopathic doctor, when my son's appendix ruptured or when I broke my leg, we immediately went to the emergency room, grateful for the doctors and surgeons that took care of us and provided pain medication and excellent service at that moment.

However, when it comes to chronic issues of the body, especially pain or autoimmune disease the allopathic doctors have few answers other than trying an array of prescription medicines to alleviate one's symptoms. I have visited with several physicians over the years and in frustration they agree with this opinion. Many have expressed to me their disappointment after years of schooling and training, of not being able to cure or often times even help the myriads of our current population that seek out their help for ongoing and progressing degenerate disease or pain.

Part of the problem lies in the fact that there are other systems of the body that are clearly recognized in many parts of the world that are not taught or discussed in medical schools in the United States. Therefore, these systems are overlooked when examining a patient to determine the best protocol for treating their body. In fact my experience has been that if you ask a medical doctor or often times even a chiropractic doctor if they think craniosacral therapy will help in your situation you will most likely get one of the following responses. "I imagine it will help you feel good at the moment, but I don't think it will actually help your problem." Or, "You could try it but don't expect too much." I realize these statements come from a lack of knowledge of these others systems of the body and techniques used to manipulate the function of these systems. Drawing from my sixteen years of experience I want to show you what this little known, but highly effective therapy can really do.

Chapter 1

Are You Ready To Explore Other Options?

Are you asking yourself, "Do I want to keep living in pain?" "Do I want to stay on pain medications the rest of my life?" "Is my current medical care giving me what I need?" Perhaps you haven't been able to get resolution or answers to your specific health needs. Maybe you're not comfortable with the multiple medications you're doctor has you taking and are concerned about their side effects down the road. Then let me ask you:

Do You Suffer From:

- Chronic headaches or backaches,
- Fibromyalgia or Chronic Fatigue,
- Chronic Ear Pain,
- Or random unexplained body aches?

Do You Find Yourself:

- Clenching or grinding your teeth,
- Feeling stressed or burned out,
- Having a loss of desire or frustrated.
- Tossing and turning at night instead of sleeping soundly?

Have You:

- Put on weight or struggled with weight issues,
- Chronic reoccurring injuries
- Been diagnosed with an auto-immune disease,
- Been feeling out-of-control of your life?

Ben, a 50 year old male, working in an executive position for a technology company had been referred to me through a friend of his. He suffered from severe headaches several times a month. They would come on first as an overwhelming fatigue, followed by a low grade tension in the base of his skull. This would progress up the side of his head to just above the left ear and eventually settling into his left eye. His eye would tear and swell and become extremely painful, "until I want to yank it right out of the socket". The tension at the base of the skull would gradually seep into the neck and shoulder until it hurt to even turn his head or lift his arm. "Once they start I know I'm in for a bad ride for three days, no matter what. I can take medication, or not, I can rest, or not, I can get a massage, or not....it doesn't matter. Until those three days have passed my pain level will go – on a scale of 1 to 10 –

to *15*. It'll stay that way for most of a day, then drop off drastically and be totally gone by the end of the third day."

Anyone who has suffered from migraines will recognize most of this cycle. However, with migraines, often if it is caught in the early stages, medication or sleep will way lay them. But Ben was emphatic this was not the case. He had a CT scan, and MRI, tried migraine medications and even had a sleep study done to track brain waves over a period of time. But all tests came up negative and medication didn't help. He did admit that he was under a great deal of stress with pressures at work. It was not unusual for him to work 10 or 12 hour days when a project was in full swing or meeting a deadline. His wife worked and so he felt guilty when he wasn't able to come home and help her with their two sons.

"If I have to continue with this much longer, I will lose my job and, well" shaking his head and looking away his voice trailed to a desperate whisper, "I just don't know that I," he paused then proceeded shaking his head, "I can't continue with life if it is going to be like this." His voice caught in his throat, a red embarrassed flush crept from his starched white shirt collar moving up his throat and face. The muscles in his jaw tightened as he tried to control his frustration and feeling of utter helplessness.

Lindsay came walking into my office, a slight young woman in her early 30s. She was definitely underweight by perhaps 10-15 pounds. Looking at her I saw a perfectly put together fashion picture. But what was odd was she seemed like a one dimensional picture, rather than a living breathing person.

I welcomed her with a smile and a hand shake as I introduced myself. The smile was returned, the polite words and expressions, but they were hollow. It was haunting to encounter this shell of a person who had a name and a history but so little substance. She had been referred to me by her naturopathic doctor to see what I could do about her constant random body pain.

As I reviewed her medical history from the previous five years I saw that she had been diagnosed with fibromyalgia, irritable bowel syndrome, and extensive food and environmental allergies. She had also been diagnosed with depression but her doctor felt that was a response to the fibro and IBS. Her irritable bowel syndrome coupled with the resulting depression was believed to be the cause of her continual weight loss. She had originally been prescribed Paxil for her depression and fibromyalgia symptoms and Alosetron for the IBS. However, due to the side effects and safety concerns with Alosetron, even though it seemed to help, the doctor took her off it after just a few months.

Then I began to explore Lindsay's experience with the prescription medications, asking her questions. She told me she had chosen to go off the Paxil since she hadn't felt any relief of her pain, her insomnia worsened and she didn't have the increase in energy the doctor had hoped to achieve. The doctors had suggested they try Zoloft but she had declined. They told her there was nothing more they could do for her. She said she was so discouraged, hurting all the time, and couldn't eat because everything went straight through her, and now her doctor basically had told her she would have to learn to live with it or try different medications. No wonder Lindsay felt depressed.

At that point, like so many people today, Lindsay turned to the internet for help. She found a discussion board for IBS and through reading it found that many had found help with a naturopathic doctor who looked at the body as a whole, rather than as individual diagnosis. She began to ask around and when she had heard the same name three times, she decided to call him. He was helping her with the IBS and allergies but referred her to me for the pain issues which were not resolving. We needed to find some answers for her and give her hope.

11

These kinds of pleas for help are not new to me or anyone else who works in the chronic pain or disease field.

The Epidemic Of Chronic Pain

Chronic pain has reached epidemic levels in the United States alone. According to the American Pain Foundation an estimated **50 million** Americans suffer with persistent pain each year. If you add one to two loved ones for each of those people, you realize that pain is directly affecting **100 – 150 million** people a year. That is nearly half the population.

The American Alliance of Cancer Pain Initiatives (AACPI) estimates 1 in 3 Americans lose more than 20 hours of sleep each month due to pain.

Like Ben's case, The National Headache Foundation reports that headaches are the most common type of pain and that approximately **$50 billion** per year is lost in industries due to absenteeism and medical expenses related to headaches.

Generalized chronic pain is the second leading cause of medically related work absenteeism, resulting in more than **$50 million** lost in work days missed in a given year. This statistic comes from the American Pain Society.

The National Institutes of Health estimates up to **23.5 million** Americans suffer from autoimmune disease and that the prevalence is rising. They have identified 80-100 different autoimmune diseases and suspect at least 40 additional diseases of having an autoimmune basis.

These studies show how significant the problem of chronic pain (and chronic illness which creates pain) is to our society today. And these studies don't even address the issues that these chronic conditions play in interfering with social relationships, family life and self-esteem.

It is astounding to realize that research done by the National Institute Of Mental Health shows that 1 in 4 or 25% of our population suffer with some form of diagnosed disorder. These disorders include, anxiety disorders, attention deficit disorder, eating disorders, autism, mood disorders, and personality disorders. Notice that these statistics are of diagnosed cases, which means the numbers are actually much higher.

The Good News

There is good news though for those of you who suffer from chronic conditions from which you have not received answers and also for those of you who have thought you would be relegated to taking medications for the rest of your life while dealing with their undesirable side effects. There are therapies that have been proven to make a significant difference in people's lives. These therapies have been around for hundreds of years but in the United States have only recently been unburied or gradually brought into people's awareness.

The first steps to understanding your pain and moving through it is *opening your mind to new possibilities and old but innovative avenues of arriving at the new healthier you.* The human body was not created to self-destruct but to self-heal. We see living proof of this concept each time we cut ourselves and the cut heals over forming a scab and eventually heals completely. Sometime without even leaving a scar or any trace of the wound. The same is true with a broken bone. It has the ability to heal itself with very little intervention from the outside. However, the common thread in the body being able to heal itself is the necessity of creating an appropriate and therapeutic environment for the healing to take place. In the case of the cut, if the wound is too deep it will necessitate creating an environment cleansed from debris or germs and then closed so that the tissue is close enough that the body can fill in the space with fibragen tissues. So the doctor uses stitches to close the wound and create the appropriate environment. In the case of the broken bone, setting it and immobilizing it with a cast or splint for a period of time creates a therapeutic environment. This type of environment is known as a healthy physiological environment.

The Energetic Body

There is another component, however, to the healing environment of the body that has been a little slower in being understood or studied. Whether you know, understand or believe the Eastern Medicine component of energy medicine or not; the bottom line is our bodies are energy. Even Western Medicine uses the energetic systems of the body as a tool to gather information for diagnosis when they administer EKGs or EEGs on a patient. So let's explore the energy concept in this next section.

For hundreds of years Traditional Chinese Medicine has understood and touted the importance of a life force they call "Qi". They believe this force needs to be present and flowing throughout the body in order for healing and health to exist. In India they have revered the healing forces of this same energy known to them as Prana or Chi. Such "energy" is often seen as a continuum that unites body and mind. It is sometimes conceived of as a universal life force running within and between all things, the natural energy of self.

This energetic environment sometimes known as spiritual energy is closely associated with the metaphor of life as breath. The words it is known by around the world, qi, prana, spirit, light of Christ, or Holy Ghost, are all related in their respective languages and contexts to the verb 'to breathe' or referring to the movement of breath in the body or the bodies vitality. Each country or spiritual background may have a slight variation on the meaning but at the core it is what makes you, you.

Meeting The Headwind

The conflict in our modern society since the emergence of Allopathic medicine has been that scientists and doctors have felt there is not enough scientific based research to explain this energetic environment of the body and its affect on health and healing. However, bioenergetics is a formalized branch of biochemistry that has been formed to study the effects of energy flow through the living systems. (Not just humans but all things living.) In their research they study thousands of different cellular processes such as cellular respiration and the many other metabolic processes that lead to production and utilization of energy within the living system.

Growth, development and metabolism within our bodies are some of the phenomena resulting from the energy formed and used within our bodies. Science recognizes that energy is fundamental to our processes. The ability of our body to harness the energy it can produce and use in metabolic pathways is widely accepted in the scientific world. In fact, we survive only because of the body's ability to create, harness and exchange energy within and without itself. Much of this energy process is due to ionic (positively and negatively) charged chemicals and particles in and around our cells. The electromagnetic field created around these processes and the interaction or flow of field of energy is what we call the bodies energetic Qi, or Prana, or Spirit.

Because all living things have Qi each of us can affect or be affected by other living organism's electromagnetic field. Think of a baby who begins to cry when someone else comes into the room who is in intense pain or stressed or angry. Even though the person has no immediate interaction with the baby, the baby senses the change and becomes nervous or stressed. This same interchange of energy is what has been researched with the higher growth rates of plants when people talk or sing to them.

Another function of energy that each of us experience each time we walk outside into the sun is the phenomenon of sunlight being converted to Vitamin D in our bodies. It is the frequency of energy, in this case sunlight, entering our body creating a chemical reaction that results in the creation of vitamin D. The same is true when we get a sun tan. In this case the frequency of energy creates the chemical reaction of creating melanin, which is an antioxidant. It is produced when the frequency of energy that is hitting our bodies is too high and our body is trying to protect itself from the damage being done. (This info comes from Dr. David Schmidt, scientist hired by US government to design ways to keep submarine crews alive longer in event of an accident and special op teams alert and functioning at an optimum level for longer periods of time.)

Other research besides bioenergetics was done years ago by a German physician named Reinhold Voll. In our body, there are areas along channels of energy or meridians that have a different electrical conductivity than in other areas along the line or channel and these are called acupuncture points which connect all the systems of the body together. These points and channels of energy correspond to specific areas, systems and organs of the body. Most of these channels have control end points located on the ears, hands and feet. In the 1950's Dr. Voll, developed an electrical device called a Dermatron to measure and monitor the conductivity of energy on acupuncture points. Dr. Voll's device had a meter with a scale that went from 0 to 100, with a reading of 50 representing optimal energy coming off the point indicating good health. If the acupuncture point measured above 55 it would indicate too much energy was coming off of the point and inflammation was occurring in the system or organs dictated by that point; below 45 would indicate low energy coming from a point creating a degenerated condition. Currently in many parts of the world, a form of this electrical device is used in doctor's offices, hospitals and clinics to aid the health practitioner to determine the energetic condition of the different systems of the body and to improve the condition.

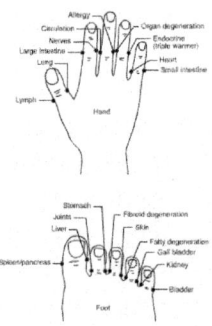

The levels of life force - Chi / Prana / qi - in our bodies have an impact on our overall inherent healing ability. Qi helps to nourish the structure, organs and systems of the body, supporting them in their vital functions and contributing to the healthy growth and renewal of cells as shown by the readings on Dr. Voll's machine.

The amount of energy created and/or absorb on a cellular level is not constant, and can depend on many factors, so we don't always sufficiently replenish our energy. If this happens over some time our energetic body can become too depleted, and this is when we become weaker and more susceptible to illness, the ageing process and even physical death, because our Qi, or life force, that which defines us as living beings is out of balance.

This means that when our Qi is at a healthy level and flowing freely around our whole body, in and around our cells, in our fluids, along our meridians, we feel healthy, strong, fit and full of energy. We also feel confident, ready to enjoy life and take on its challenges, and are much less likely to become ill. However if our Qi is low, or if there is a restriction or blockage in its flow, our cellular process suffers, we feel weak, tired, listless and lethargic, and are much more vulnerable to illness.

There are several techniques and therapies to move or manipulate a person's energy. Dedicated scientists, psychologists, bioenergetic researchers and health practitioners are finding healing potential by understanding more clearly how important this energetic information-based medicine process is to our body's health.

These therapies, known as alternative or complimentary therapies, fall under the umbrella of what is now referred to as *energy medicine.* One of the primary differences between allopathic medicine and energy medicine is that allopathic medicine has become extremely specialized. They look at your cardiac system, or your immune system, or your reproductive system or your nervous system and proceed to optimize its function. In energy medicine there is an understanding that your body is a whole entity. You cannot divide it up into systems, as each system functions in relationship to another. Even your mind and thought processes of the brain affects the function of the internal workings of your entire body.

When a soccer team is losing because the other team is constantly scoring goals, the coach doesn't just replace the goalie. He has to fix the entire defensive team so the ball only gets to the goalie when the other defenses break down. Remember our example of your checking account. You have to fix the core issue, not the symptom.

Another key concept in complimentary medicine is that the words "diagnosis" and "treatment" have a different meaning than they do in conventional medicine. In conventional medicine you diagnose and treat an illness. In energy medicine, you assess where the energy system needs attention and correct the energy disturbances. Physical symptoms may be a clue, but they are not the focus. For instance, the same stomach ache might be traced to an imbalance in the heart meridian in one person, in the liver meridian in another, and in the stomach meridian in a third. The same physical symptoms can reflect many different kinds of problems in your energy system and call for diverse kinds of attention.

19

Complimentary medicine takes into consideration your spiritual and emotional thought processes. This type of medicine understands how your heart longs for a different existence; one where your body is functioning as optimally as possible. Your heart wanting to trust that your body can get you to that point. Your heart and your mind are one entity. Your pain is not just physical. Your heart and soul long for the carefree days of movement without thought, but with the physical pain you feel as though your body has abandoned your heart leaving it shattered on the floor of your existence. Nevertheless the heart and body are one as sure as the stars and moon are in mutual existence each night. Your heart will fail to flourish without the rest of your body. Your body cannot progress back to health without its heart.

The body represents the conscious part of your existence; the soul/heart is the unconscious....let's have them work together just as two partners who purchase a failing company and create a business plan that will meet their common goals and desires of success begin to work together with a rhythm that is uniquely theirs. Let complimentary medicine be the plan to bring your heart and body together for a successfully healthy you.

You are not alone in your pain, your body's dysfunction or your frustrations. You are among millions who are looking beyond allopathic medicine for answers. More than 80 million Americans use complementary and alternative medicine (CAM) every year and the ranks are growing. CAM is a group of diverse medical and health care systems, practices, and products that, even though they are not presently considered to be part of conventional medicine, are making a significant difference for people suffering from chronic pain, disease, and disorders. According to research done at Stanford University's Complimentary and Alternative Medicine Program, more than 68% of American adults have used at least one kind of CAM therapy in any given year.

Chapter 2

What is CST (Craniosacral Therapy)

One therapy of alternative medicine used for treating chronic pain and disease that I would like to introduce you to is Craniosacral Therapy (pronounced **krey**-nee-*uh*l **sey**-kr*uh*l).

We are all familiar with the cardiovascular and respiratory rhythms of the human body. Like these, there is another rhythmic system of the body called the Craniosacral system. It has a rate and a rhythm of its own that influences many body functions that helps relieve pain and create optimal functioning of the body's other systems. The craniosacral system consists of the membranes and cerebrospinal fluid that surrounds and protects the brain and the spinal cord. It extends from the bones of the skull, face and mouth, which

21

is the cranium, therefore cranial, to the sacrum or tailbone, therefore sacral, and the spine that lies between.

This area is what houses the central nervous system of the body. All nerves of the body originate from the area encompassing the craniosacral system. The cranial nerves originate in the brain while the spinal nerves begin in the spine. These nerves send out messages from the brain dictating all functions of the body, whether it be the senses of the body, organ function, or muscle function or any other action in the body. This is why it is extremely important that this system of your body is operating at its highest level.

Research in the area of generalized pain and dysfunction has led to the development of this non-invasive light touch therapy known as craniosacral therapy. In the early 1900s an osteopathic physician by the name of William G. Sutherland began the exploration of the body's mechanical function. Osteopathic physicians, like allopathic physicians can choose any specialty, prescribe drugs, perform surgeries, and practice medicine. However, they bring the additional benefit of osteopathic manipulative techniques for the purposes of diagnoses and treatment of their patients. Osteopathic medicine first developed from the 1870s onwards in America, under the initial inspiration and guidance of Andrew Taylor Still (1828-1917), who claimed to have discovered a revolutionary system of healing and an associated therapeutic philosophy. This system of healing was based upon two related principal elements; **that the healthy body already contained all the relevant necessities for maintaining itself, and that it thus did not need the drug-based remedies of the day.** Osteopathic medicine's philosophy that improper alignment of tissues produces an inclination to various types of diseases by affecting the neurological system as well as the circulation of blood and body fluids which are essential to good health.

Dr. Sutherland took Dr. Still's philosophy and built upon it. He believed the body was a living breathing entity. He based his further beliefs on these basic principles:

- Motion at the cranial sutures, the joints linking the 26 bones of the skull
- "Expansion and contraction" of the hemispheres of the brain
- Motion of the membranes covering the brain and spinal cord
- A fluid wave within the cerebrospinal fluid that bathes the brain and spinal cord
- Involuntary, subtle motion of the sacrum (tailbone).

He did several rudimentary experiments to prove that the bones of the skull are not fused into one body as is taught in traditional medical schools, but that the bones move from their sutures. He realized that all the studies that had been done previously which led to the belief of a solid skull were done on cadavers whose bones were set in rigor mortis and moved as one bone. So he did his experiments on living people. He used basic sonar equipment as a means of recording the movement of the bones in the skull. He called this rhythmic movement of the bones and membranes 'The Primary Respiration' because he felt it was perhaps the most essential mechanism of human life. But only a small percentage of osteopathic or medical doctors accepted his work, even though he had a successful track record of treating a myriad of symptoms in his patients. Until his death in 1954 he received criticism for his treatment of patients and his publications.

With his death, much of his work slid into oblivion with only a few dedicated supporters quietly following in his footsteps. Dr. Robert Fulford was one of those faithful followers. He graduated from Kansas City School of Osteopathy and Surgery in 1941 and soon after met and studied with Dr. Sutherland. He said that Dr. Sutherland always taught "to dig on" beyond what you have learned in school. Dr. Fulford did just that, pioneering the introduction of alternative and energetic medicine in the context of osteopathic medicine. Beginning in the nineteen forties, he developed methods of working in the "energy body" too resolve chronic complaints which had an energetic, emotional, or spiritual component. Dr. Fulford was one of the first physicians to emphasize publicly the idea that "thoughts are things" and integrated the use of intention into his practice of manual adjustments on his patients.

Another osteopathic doctor, Dr. John Upledger was assisting in a back surgery one day while doing his residency, when he actually observed the rhythmic movement of the craniosacral system. At the time, none of his colleagues or his medical text books could explain to him what he had observed. Two years later, still searching for answers Dr. Upledger attended a course that had originally been developed by Dr. Sutherland. The startling facts that Dr. Upledger learned in that course about the movement of cranial bones was fascinating to him. This made sense to Upledger when he combined it with the odd pulsing rhythm he had experienced during the earlier spinal surgery. He theorized that there must be a sort of hydraulic system inside the craniosacral system. So he set out to prove his theory.

In 1975 he obtained funds to study this theory and joined a team of osteopathic physicians like himself at the Osteopathic College at Michigan State University as a clinical researcher and professor of biomechanics. There he led his team through tests done with x-ray films of living skulls that showed cranial motion. These motions were detected and measured using sensitive instruments. They were finally able to document the influence of Dr. Sutherland's theory of the craniosacral system. For the first time they were now also able to explain the function of this system. Dr. Upledger then went on to develop and test how light touch manual therapy could be used to evaluate and manipulate this system to treat malfunctions in the body. He titled his therapy Craniosacral Therapy.

As mentioned earlier, all body functions from the production of cells to the contracting of muscles comes from nerves either originating in the brain or in the spine. Those nerves originating from the brain are known as cranial nerves and those from the spine, spinal nerves. Because these nerves all originate in the craniosacral system this therapy is able to influence all systems of the body making it highly effective in treating the whole body, not just one specific area or issue.

The cerebral spinal fluid is inside the spinal column. It resonates up the spinal column, through a membrane system, to the top of the brain, pauses and then descends back down the column while partially being reabsorbed into the blood. When the fluid is partially reabsorbed the body senses the decrease in pressure within the column and generates production of more fluid causing an increase in the pressure which starts the fluid rising up the column again similar to a partial hydraulic system. The purpose of this rise and fall is thought to be twofold. First the cerebral spinal fluid is continually flushing between all the brain cells and the spinal cord cells. Secondly, it is rinsing and nourishing the cranial and spinal nerves. This rhythmic pattern of creation/rise and re-absorption/fall goes on in a healthy person all day, every day. However, due to birth trauma, emotional trauma, illness, injury, and a multitude of other causal effects this rhythm can be distorted or slowed down causing toxins to remain in the brain and spinal column causing a misfiring of the nerve messages coming from the cranial or spinal nerves. This misfiring of the nerves is due to the cerebral spinal fluid not getting to the nerves, rinsing them and nourishing them or cleansing or feeding the cells.

The therapist cannot actually feel the cerebral spinal fluid moving but what they are trained to do is to feel the body's response to the movement. As the fluid rises the body expands slightly moving into *extension* and when the fluid descends and is reabsorbed the body returns to neutral or into *flexion*. It is very much like observing a person breathing. As they breath in air the body expands to make

25

room for the air, and as they breath out, dispelling the air, the body returns to its neutral state. This rhythmic movement of breathing is known as our respiratory rhythm, the rise and fall of the cerebral fluid is called the craniosacral rhythm or CSR. This extension and flexion pattern of the cranial system is what the therapist learns to palpate. She wants to be able to feel the extension and flexion or expansion and return to neutral going on symmetrically throughout the entire body.

Keep in mind that the body is governed by the central nervous system (the cranial nerves and the spinal nerves). So as the cerebral spinal fluid moves past a nerve it will cause a response (extension when the fluid is rising and flexion as it is descending and being reabsorbed) to the areas that are governed by that nerve. Such as the nerves coming out of the lower spine area (Lumbar vertebrae L1=L5) govern what happens in the pelvic region and the legs. So if the therapist wants to observe what the fluid is doing in that area he/she could place her hands lightly on the hips, legs, ankles or feet and observe the CSR. Likewise, if the therapist wants to know what is happening with the upper spine (Cervical vertebrae C1=C7) which dictates function to neck, shoulder, lungs, stomach he/she could palpate the shoulders, the rib cage or the diaphragm/stomach area.

Another important part of Craniosacral Therapy is the use of techniques to remove or correct the lesions or restrictions that are causing the system to not function optimally. One of these techniques is Fascial Release. Fascia, is a three dimensional webbing that exists throughout our bodies. It is what keeps our organs suspended so they don't fall to our legs each time we stand up. It runs around and through our soft tissues, such as muscles, around our veins and arteries and surrounds and weaves through the brain.

Each of you have made or witnessed a bed being made. As you pull one corner of the sheet around and under the mattress and move to the opposite corner to do the same, you will often see wrinkles in the sheet. So you move to yet another corner stretching and straightening the sheet. Finally pulling on the last corner you attempt to remove all wrinkles by making a final adjustment to the sheet. Now it lies flat against the mattress. Well the same thing happens inside our bodies.

Through injury, illness, inflammation, over use, under use and poor nutrition this flexible webbing becomes more like a solid sheath than the mobile supple webbing it is meant to be. This webbing can begin to pull and tug critical bones, joints and organs from their intended locations creating compensation patterns not unlike the wrinkles in the sheets when we first start making up the bed. According to John F. Barnes, PT this tugging motion can also put a tensile pressure equal to 2000 pounds per square inch on sensitive tissues and organs causing extraordinary pain. He also reminds us that this tension in the fascia will not show up on ordinary medical tests such as x-rays, CT scans and MRI scans. Because it is one continuous structure from the top of your head to your toes a wrinkle or bound up area in one area of your body can be felt in a totally different location. (Remember the bed sheet analogy.) Therefore it is the therapist's job to locate and smooth out those wrinkles in the fascial and membrane systems of the body to allow the body to return to its normal healthy environment. This means the therapist may not work in the area you are actually feeling the pain or discomfort in but will go to a primary area of fascial dysfunction and begin smoothing and unraveling the fascial from that point.

These fascial restrictions, the compensation your body has made because of them, or the inflammation or the dysfunction of organs they've contributed to may be part of the reason the craniosacral system is not functioning optimally.

Another therapy used in conjunction with craniosacral therapy is acupressure. Acupressure is an ancient healing art using fingers to apply small amounts of pressure to strategic points on the surface of the skin to encourage the body's natural healing ability. These key points on the body's surface, called acupressure or acupuncture points, are especially sensitive to bioelectrical impulses in the body. These points carry the chi or ki to specific parts of the body. When stimulated either with pressure from the therapists hand, needles or heat they help the body release endorphins, which are the neuro-chemicals that relieve pain and make us feel happy and relaxed. As a result the pain is blocked or diminished, the flow of blood and oxygen are sent to the area being stimulated as well as along the meridian or pathway to which that specific point is connected.

Many of the acupuncture meridians either end or begin or interface with the craniosacral system. Moving along the base of the skull, where most people tend to hold their stress are the points for the triple warmer, gallbladder, bladder, and the governing vessel. Let's look at each of these points and their accompanying meridian to see how they can affect a person's CSR.

The governing vessel meridian runs from the top of your head to the end of your tail bone carrying the body's energy to and through the craniosacral system. By balancing two points on this meridian, one at the base of the skull and one that lies over the first and second cervical vertebra, headaches at the base of the skull, especially with neck stiffness, upper cervical pain and restricted neck rotation can be helped by relaxing the associated muscles. This is important so that the occipital bone, the bone compromising the lower third of the back of the skull, can move freely and in sync with the movement of the tailbone.

The triple warmer, sometimes called triple heater or triple burner, regulates metabolism by balancing the thyroid and the adrenal (stress) glands. It also affects the immune

28

system, but its interaction with craniosacral therapy is mostly related to its metabolic function. Balancing this meridian will help reduce stress induced anxiety, addressing panic, stress, trauma, energy drain and helping hyperactive children all of which can reduce the function of the craniosacral system.

The Gallbladder meridian's chi is easily influenced by a person's emotional state. Psychological pressure and stress, such as anger, irritation, feelings of being annoyed and frustration weaken the flow of the energy in the gallbladder and bile, and also in the liver. It is closely related to eye problems, migraine and tinnitus (ringing in the ear). Disturbances of the gallbladder and the bile ducts are frequently the primary cause of many chronic health problems such as migraine, headache, eye diseases, ear and nose problems, such as sinusitis creating a disturbance in the craniosacral system.

The bladder point and its meridian are considered important in dealing with issues related to head, eyes and sinus. However, according to Traditional Chinese Medicine a close connection exists between the bladder and the kidney meridian. Therefore the bladder meridian has a special relationship with the pelvic area. This is critical for cranial work since the pelvic bones must move in synchrony with the head bones to keep the rocking, pumping motion of the cranial system moving. If there are disturbances in the pelvic region it could slow or stop the CSR.

Balancing

By balancing these critical acupressure points at the base of the client's skull the therapist can begin to resolve many issues that could be playing a role in optimizing the craniosacral system.

The client's emotional well-being intricately affects the CSR. Therefore Emotional Release Therapy is another critical adjunct to craniosacral therapy. Have you ever had a physical injury that continued to plague you even after the injury seemingly healed? This is not unusual. Even when alternative healing practices such as acupuncture, acupressure, craniosacral therapy, or massage are used the pain or illness returns after a short period of time, or at the same time each year. When this happens it is almost always a sign that there is an emotional imbalance or memory pattern associated with the injury or illness.

The cells of the muscle tissue have memory. This is another area of debate between alternative therapists and convention medical professionals. But it is agreed among all that there are neural pathways in and from the brain that will give the muscles this sense of muscle memory. Whether it is the pathways alone, or in conjunction with the actual cellular memory isn't as important as the effect this phenomena has on the physical body. An athlete is trained over and over again under various conditions to make a shot, complete a pass, catch a pass, drive a golf ball 250 feet, etc. so that at the moment they have to perform this precise task under whatever circumstances their muscle memory will take over and perform without normal step by step brain processing. The same is true with musicians. The practicing of playing an instrument over and over produces the memory in the extremities of the body as well as the brain so that the musician can play it automatically without the brain needing to process each note individually.

This same muscle memory process is what allows trained Navy Seal members to be able to control emotions and pain so that it will not affect their performance as it would the typical person. Their bodies are conditioned to use the skills and responses developed through muscle memory under extremely stressful and unexpected conditions. Muscle memory is a very powerful tool allowing the mind to dictate the physical body.

Just as we can train the muscles to perform the task we desire or teach the body to desensitize the sensation of pain the same process can happen subconsciously when we experience a strong emotional reaction to a physical event. Therefore, in the future when any event triggers a similar emotion the original physical reaction in the body will be experienced. For our discussion here, that sense would usually be physical pain or illness. When this happens it can slow down or even shut down the CSR depending on the degree of emotional/physical reaction the client is experiencing.

Most people have heard of a polygraph test, more commonly known as a lie detector test. What this test does is measures and records several physiological responses, such as blood pressure, respiratory rhythm, eye dilation, skin conductivity and pulse. When the person taking the test is asked a question they are comfortable with, the different rhythms in their body remain unchanged. However, when asked a question they feel compelled to lie about the physical responses mentioned above will speed up or spike. You are probably wondering what this has to do with the CSR. As I mentioned previously, the CSR is another biological rhythm in our body. It too can act as an indicator to give valuable information. When the client is asked a question and the answer is yes the CSR will stop, but if the answer is no it will speed up. I use this technique to determine where the emotions are being held in the body, the surrounding circumstances of the event experienced as well as the primary emotion being held there. Through a series of questions asked while observing the CSR this information is made available so that the client can process the emotion and release it from the physical body neutralizing the affect the deeply felt and held emotion can have on the physical body in the future.

31

This technique works wonderfully with people who experienced the trauma at an age prior to being able to verbalize what they experienced or felt or when the event was too traumatic to be able to verbalize it (as with PTSD as we will discuss in the case history in chapter 7) because the body will provide the information needed rather than the conscious intellect. Then once the information is gained it can be released, often times without deep analysis or drama. The most typical emotions found with emotional release are fear, anger, hatred, frustration, loneliness, guilt or humiliation. Please note that the events leading to or being held in the tissues does not have to be a major traumatic event but something perceived as traumatic or unexpected that elicits a strong emotion.

Sensing - Intuitive

I've introduced you to the linear, functional aspects of craniosacral therapy and some of its adjunct therapies. But there is another facet which is much more difficult to put into words. If a therapist truly believes in the concept that a person's body fully knows what it needs to heal itself then it is important that the therapist not get in the way of that healing mechanism with a preconceived notion of what needs to happen in the person's body. I tend to ask very few questions of my client's health history as I would prefer the body tell me its history. The client lies on the table, fully clothed while I sit down. Placing my hands on a specific part of their body I need to open my mind and my heart and simply listen to what their body is telling me. That may sound rather odd to you, but I am simply the facilitator helping their body move down the path toward wholeness. When I give my hands the opportunity to do what your body needs, my hands often times move as if they were not really connected to me but are guided by another force. I will ask your body where I should start and then wait for the CSR to tell me. When I move my hands to that area I trust my hands to trigger the necessary response. Often the client will say, "Oh that is where it has been bothering me," or "How did you know to go there? That is where it has been hurting." A good craniosacral therapist will not try to *make* your body do something but will *assist* your body to do what it needs to do. They won't try to get your muscle to do what they want it to, but will wait for the body to dictate what needs to happen and will trust that your body will make that known. Dr. Sutherland, years ago, taught "the healing is in the stillness". This takes time to understand. This is the intuitive part of craniosacral therapy that is much harder for newcomers to the therapy to understand and become comfortable with.

I have been asked multiple times by clients, "Are you physic?" The answer is, "No." I have simply learned to be quiet, open my mind to all possibilities and then get out of the way and watch the miracles happen. It is an amazing thing to behold. I first came into this work at the suggestion of an orthodontist. I was working as a dental consultant in his office. One day after finishing up a staff meeting he asked if he could see me in his office. When I entered the office he closed the door and looking intently at me said, "You are good at what you do. But (don't you just love that word) I can tell you aren't passionate about it." My first thought was that there was a need I was not fulfilling so I asked what he would like to see me do differently. He reassured me there was nothing within the context of my consulting position he wanted me to do differently but he shared with me this thought. "I've lived long enough to know that life is too short to waste time doing something you aren't passionate about."

He then asked me what I would do if I could do anything I wanted. As a young mother, wife and professional my response was simple, "Survive". We shared a laugh and then I confessed I had no idea. He told me he had been observing me and thought I would be a great craniosacral therapist and wanted me to be trained and bring it into the dental world where it was greatly needed. Like many of you, I had never heard of craniosacral therapy. He gave me the name and telephone number of the Upledger Institute.

After completing my training and feeling rather smug about my skill level I returned to this orthodontist's office reporting in that I had finished training and felt quite comfortable going into any dentist's office and giving their patients craniosacral therapy. He was sitting behind his desk at the time. He arose, walked around to where I was standing and putting a fatherly arm around my shoulder and giving it a little squeeze he said, "You're just a babe. Give it about 10 years and you might begin to understand the work."

I was more than just a little offended by his comment and demeanor. I had worked very hard the past eighteen months. I was good at this. But now, 15 years later, I realize the wisdom in his words. It took years for me to let go of my ego and years of ingrained linear thinking so that I could get out of the way of my client's own healing power and simply provide the optimum environment so their healing could take place.

I will forever be grateful to Dr. Leo Jaegar who saw something in me, I couldn't see and who passed along such great wisdom. I love this work and after having the opportunity to be part of the healing process of hundreds of clients I have developed a passion not only for my work but for all of life. I've discovered the layered wisdom in the words, "Life is too short to waste time doing something you aren't passionate about." When you begin to feel great passion in one aspect of your life, it flows freely into other pieces like the lava flowing out of a volcano, running hot into crevices, filling you with an urgency to live each day fully and a burning desire to move on, experiencing life on a deeper more profound level than ever before.

34

These techniques and therapies I've discussed are new or little known of by many of you. The natural tendency of many people is to resist that which is unfamiliar. The familiar, whether working and producing a healthy life or not is often accepted simply because of its familiarity, rather than looking at or becoming involved in the unknown world of the unfamiliar. Look how many people stay in poor relationships, knowing and complaining that it isn't working, rather than go to counseling or ending the relationship because they fear the unknown and unfamiliar road ahead. The same is true of people in jobs they feel unhappy in or sense they are at a dead end. Rather than jump out there into the world of the "unknown" that could produce a happy and fulfilling career for them, they stay put in the security of the "familiar". You have a choice to make. The "familiar", that has not achieved a happy, healthier, pain free you or has you using multiple medications and feeling out of control of your own health, or taking a risk with the "unfamiliar" but proven techniques and therapies suggested in this book. Which will you choose? The choice is yours.

Chapter 3

Overcoming Resistance

It is my hope that this book will provide a well-marked pathway that will help you traverse from the known to the unknown, from the traditional healing model to a complimentary model of wholeness. Just as there are often broken sidewalks, or rocks along many paths there will be obstacles along this route that you will need to overcome. It is my intention to address those obstacles right up front. There is an interesting question I like to ask. *If you were packing to pursue a dream, what would you take with you and what would you leave behind?* I present this question to you, the reader, because I would imagine that you have a dream of a healthy, pain-free life or you dream of returning to the days of mobility and energy you once knew.

One of the items I would encourage you to pack in your suitcase would be *knowledge*. Another important tool is a healthy dose of *curiosity*, coupled with *open mindedness.* Also vital -- a great *support system.*

Items you will definitely want to leave behind are unawareness based on old patterns of thinking, and a closed off mindset. For sure you will want to leave behind the Nay Sayers. Those family members, friends (I use that term loosely here), and co-workers who will reassure you that IT won't work, that you are crazy to try THAT, and who don't say anything but silently shake their head or say "I wouldn't do THAT."

We've talked significantly about the first couple of items I recommended you leave behind, the unawareness based on old pattern thinking of traditional allopathic medicine versus alternative or complimentary medicine. We've also talked about opening your mind to the possibilities of a different concept of the body's energy and wholeness playing and important role in your overall wellness. We've increased your awareness. Now I would like to address the last item I recommended you leave behind, the Nay Sayers.

I remember when I first starting doing this work. I would try to explain it to people and because it was a new concept for me at the time, I had a difficult time putting it into words. That was even after I had the luxury of reading text books and going to classes. I had grown up in a traditional family were our health was turned over to the family doctor. Most of the people I knew and associated with were from the same persuasion. But I had felt the difference the CST made and I had witnessed the seemingly miraculous outcomes of the treatments so I was excited about it.

However, I found that again, as I have mentioned earlier, most people are not comfortable with the unknown and so they scoff at the mention of it. As I would talk about what I had learned or felt or witnessed, people would diminish what

I was saying. They would say there was nothing to it, or that it was crazy. Even some clients that I worked with would say, " Well it feels good, but it isn't really doing anything". They would fall asleep on the table in a state of total relaxation or their pain would go away, but they would say it couldn't have been the treatment because I didn't do enough. In other words, they didn't feel pain during the session so how could I have made any difference in their body?

Have you ever witnessed a toddler experiencing ice cream for the first time? Their first response is a shudder at the coldness in their mouth but, then when they taste the sweetness, feel the smooth creamy texture their eyes light up and their whole body responds in a sense of joy. That is how it was with me and CST. At first when I started studying it I didn't actually shudder, but my traditional, scientifically instructed brain wanted to push away from the concept of skull bones moving and fluid guidance and a touch equal to the weight of a nickel. But as I continued to learn and experience Sutherland's and eventually Upledger's teachings, I could hardly contain my excitement. Nevertheless, the more friends, family and co-workers who hadn't studied or experienced CST would diminish what I was experiencing with my clients the more I began to pull into myself. What had started as a new found excitement that I wanted to share with the world began to shrivel up like a drying sponge. It hurt profoundly to see people so closed off to something that could make such a difference in people's body's and health. I knew CST was not a cure-all….I don't believe any medication or therapy is a cure-all. But, I know without any doubt that CST *and its conjunctive therapies* can make an intensely marked difference for most people.

Part of the growing process for me and of my clients is letting go of the deeply held desire to have the acceptance of those around us in all we do. This was as true for me in my professional life as a therapist as it is for me as a person. It took a while for me to realize that in pursuing my dream to become as healthy as I could possibly be and to help my clients reach that same dream, I would have to leave the Nay Sayers behind. Or at least stop listening to their negative chatter. I, as will you, need to not only intellectualize, but have my heart accept the fact that the Nay Sayers weren't attacking me personally, although it often felt that way, but they were simply uninformed and unable to move down this particular path with me, at this moment in time.

I began to guard this new information and healing technique as a parent protects a disabled child from the cruel on lookers who whisper and shy away from something with which they are uncomfortable. I would share it only with those whom I felt would and could appreciate it and of course, my clients who came to me.

As time passed the new me that could pursue dreams and engulf myself in all aspects of my work -- from the physical, to the mental, to the emotional and intuitive became the comfortable old pair of broken-in running shoes compared to the previous narrow perspective, needing acceptance me that now felt like a restrictive tight pair of high heels or a knotted dress tie. I could still put on the high heels (or the knotted tie) and look the part when I needed to be among the Nay Sayers. But as soon as possible I would slip away, kick off the high heels and luxuriate in my comfy running shoes. This is what I mean by leaving them behind. We don't necessarily exclude them from our lives but, we know their opinions of us or what we are doing is only that, their opinion. It is something we can literally kick off, like the high heels or the knotted dress tie.

This reminds me of Braden's mother. Braden was six months old when he was brought to me by his mother. He had had three significant antibiotic resistant ear infections in his short life. He had spent almost 8 weeks of his six months, a third of his life, on antibiotics. Anyone knowing how devastating antibiotics are on the digestive system would not be surprised to know that now Braden suffered from alternating diarrhea and days of constipation. He had not gained any weight in the past month and it was believed this was due to the digestive issues. Braden's mother was being encouraged to stop nursing and put him on Soy formula to see if he would do better on that. She was totally stressed out because not only had she been dealing with a cranky baby, she had been trying to alter her dietary intake to make her milk more compatible for Braden's digestive system.

Braden's paternal grandfather was a successful internist who had studied at a highly prestigious medical school. His maternal grandmother was a retired pediatric nurse. They, of course, were both very concerned for their grandchild's health and gave all sorts of professional counsel to the mother. But all that advise, even though she tried to do it all, was not making for a healthier baby. When Braden's mother confided in a girlfriend all her frustrations and tears, her friend asked if she had considered taking him to a craniosacral therapist. She had never heard of this and asked what that person would do for Braden. Her friend gave her my name and telephone number.

The day Braden came into my office was when he was suffering from constipation, gas and blotting. He had not had a bowel movement in five days. When she would try to nurse him, he would hungrily gulp down a few swallows and then start screaming. Not only was the baby in distress but his mother was obviously very tense and nervous. I gently took the fussy baby from her and gently rocked and cooed to him. After five babies of my own, a crying baby doesn't disturb me too much. With him cuddled up on my shoulder I was able to put one hand on his head and one hand on his sacrum (tailbone) and monitor his cranial rhythm. There wasn't any rhythm. I swaddled him snuggly in a blanket because most babies don't like lying loosely on a table and put one hand under him and one hand on top of his tight and

40

bulging tummy. He immediately began to cry but I kept my voice low and steady whispering into his ear while I began loosening up the tissues of his belly. Shortly he began to calm down and eventually began to drift off to sleep. At this point I was able to cradle his head and only applying the 5 grams of pressure allowed the skull to start softening in my hands. Now I realize that statement sounds odd, but that is the sensation a therapist will feel. The head will go from feeling extremely rigid to a moveable moldable object.

Braden had significant compression at the base of his skull which was not allowing the cerebral spinal fluid to pass through easily and with full pressure. I was able to release this and then watched as the sphenoid bone, the bone that holds the eyes began to release. The sphenoid bone is very important in that it articulates with every other bone in the head. When it is jammed or torque to one side, as Braden's was, it can cause all sorts of issues, especially in an infant's small skull. The side that was torque down and back was causing pressure on the tiny ear canal so that it couldn't drain properly. His mother was watching and commented on how relaxed his facial features seemed now. I then once again cradled him in my hands, one on the back of his head, the other on his bottom and elongated the sluggish cranial rhythm that was now present.

Dr. John Upledger explains this therapy in his article that appeared in The Health Visitor in July 1994. "Recurrent ear infections, otitis media, are very common in early childhood and are suitable for treatment by cranio-sacral therapy. They arise from an accunsulation and stagnation of fluids in the middle ear, behind the ear drum, which leads to infection (often recurrent) and could result in partial or even total hearing loss. The stagnation indicates lack of proper drainage from the middle ear of the accumulated fluids, which should normally pass via the eustachian tube (or auditory tube) running from the middle ear to empty into the nasopharyngeal cavity at the back of the mouth.

Constriction of the eustachian tube may occur as a result of compression or distortion during the birth process; blockage of the tube may arise due to the accumulation of mucus. Treatment of the compressions and tensions in the surrounding area by cranio-sacral therapy will generally remove the constrictions, clear the obstruction, and ensure the free drainage of fluids. Successful treatment relieves the immediate symptoms, restores proper hearing, and therefore proper learning and speech development."

He then goes on to explain in the same article why cranial therapy worked so effectively and swiftly on Braden for his colic digestive issues. To treat most cases of colic or colic-like conditions, the craniosacral therapist concentrates on the principal areas: the cranial base and the solar plexus region (the upper abdominal area). The first, the cranial base, concerns the occipital bone and its relationship with the atlas - vertebra (CI). The cranial base is the area most susceptible to compression and distortion during the birth process, due to its location and the direction of the pressure exerted on this area by the baby's passage through the birth canal. This houses the area where the vagus nerve, or nerve X passes. This provides the main parasympathetic nerve supply to most of the digestive system; its compression can lead to over-stimulation of the nerve, causing persistent spasm of the digestive organs and, consequently, colic."

I explained to his mother that infants are amazingly resilient and that he would probably only need one or two more visits. I needed to work inside his mouth to free up some restrictions in there to help him to suckle better but felt we had done enough for that day. If there had been a strain on neck and mouth/jaw these nerves may become inflamed and irritated making sucking and feeding problematic. Many babies with colic are often suffering from irritation of the nerves of the neck and mouth. These babies have difficulty in latching on to the mother's breast or a bottle and will only use part of their mouths to suck, gulp the milk and pull suddenly off the breast or away from the bottle.

I also gave her copies of research that had been done in the U.S., Canada, Europe and other developed nations citing a decrease in the incidence and severity of diarrhea, lower respiratory infections, ear infections, urinary tract infections, and allergic diseases as stated in multiple issues of the *Journal of Pediatrics* in 1992, 1993, 1994, and 1997. I encouraged her to continue nursing and not stop and switch to soy formula yet, but to give the craniosacral therapy a chance to work. She agreed and scheduled a second appointment two days later.

Braden's mother called me the next day to tell me that Braden had a normal bowel movement a couple of hours after his appointment the previous day and again that morning. He seemed happier and was sleeping better, but still struggling with nursing. I considered this great news. Then she followed that report with the news that she needed to cancel his next appointment. I told her we needed to stay on top of Braden's healing response and shouldn't let too much time go between appointments. I then asked when she could next bring him in. She hesitated and said she didn't think she would be bringing him back. I was shocked since Braden had responded so well to our first session. I reiterated to her that I felt it was important to continue therapy since Braden still had a few things we needed to deal with to help him start thriving again. She didn't respond to this. So I asked if she would be more comfortable if I referred her to someone else. She quickly assured me she was delighted with how caring I had been with Braden and that wasn't the problem.

"Then what is the problem?" I asked with sincere concern.

"Well, it is just that my family thinks this is ummm, well..." she trailed off.

"They don't understand it or have never heard of it, so they are uncomfortable with it." I finished for her.

"Yes. I'm really sorry."

She then went on to tell me about the professions of her mother and father-in-law and that they probably knew more than she did as a first time mother. In my early years of doing this work this would most likely have upset me, but I've learned everyone is on their own journey and it wasn't fair to this young mother to express my feelings about the closed mindedness of her family.

"I understand completely. I've seen this before. But I want to ask you, have the treatments that they have recommended worked to make Braden healthier?" I asked.

"No. It's like I told you yesterday. Nothing has seemed to work for more than a few days and then he is back to being miserable."

"Then what do you have to lose in trying this for at least a few days? I know it is difficult to go against the wishes of your family. But can you at least try this for a week for Braden's sake and if it isn't working then agree to try the next thing they are recommending? You are his mother. Because of that you know in your heart what is best for him, and I will honor whatever that decision is, as long as it is your decision and not someone else's."

"I feel like this worked. I watched his reaction and response as you worked on him. And I see how much calmer and content he is today than he's been since we brought him home with us. But I don't know if I can tell them that. Maybe you could talk to them." She added hopefully.

"I would be happy to answer any questions they have, but it is important that you realize this is your child. I think you can tell them you're bringing him back and then invite them to join you tomorrow if they want to ask me questions."

I wanted to empower this young mother as much as possible. I wanted her to learn about the power of standing up for what you want and still loving those who doubt you or your decision. I wanted her to understand "leaving behind the Nay Sayers."

She brought Braden in the following day, alone. No one wanted to join her. I told her how proud I was of her for standing up for her motherly intuition. I proceeded to treat Braden's mouth, release the cranial base a little more to enhance his CSR and lightly manipulate the shoulders. I didn't need to see him again as he didn't have any more ear infections and by adding probiotics to both her and Braden's diet the digestive system balanced out and his bowel movements became normal. With these enhancements in his health and him being able to suckle happily he began to gain weight and progress normally.

Because young children tumble and fall I recommend seeing them every 4-6 months unless issues arise before that time. Each time I saw Braden, I noticed how much more confident his mother was in her mothering skills. I congratulated her on this accomplishment.

Chapter 4

Therapeutic Touch

Today, we find ourselves moving toward a faceless, non-touch society. We spend most of our time either talking on a telephone, emailing or blogging on a computer or sending a quick text message. Too often it can be days between meaningful face to face conversations where we might actually shake hands, hug or give someone a reassuring squeeze of the shoulder.

Spending more time at the computer, in our cars commuting, in the office, or on business travel, we have increased stress and have fewer opportunities for physical contact. Even when people are face-to-face, concerns about sexual harassment and inappropriate touching can make us overly cautious and reluctant to touch each other. As a result, many of us may find ourselves starved for that ordinary, casual touch, one that simply says, "I care."

In recent years, researchers have begun to focus on the often more subtle kind of wordless communication: physical touch. Momentary touches, whether an exuberant high five, a warm hand on the shoulder, or even a creepy touch to the arm — can communicate an even wider range of emotion than gestures or expressions, and sometimes do so more quickly and accurately than words.

"Touch is the first language we learn," says Dacher Keltner, a professor of psychology at the University of California, Berkeley. He adds, "Touch remains our richest means of emotional expression throughout life. The evidences are stacking up quickly that touch makes a huge difference in development, participation, self-esteem, and healing."

Many studies have been done on the unhealthy effects that result from *lack of touch* or *inappropriate touch*. Sadly, it seems these studies and the situations that drive them are what most people are familiar with, because they make the headlines: *Clergyman Investigated For Sexual Abuse; Kindergarten Teacher Accused of Physical Misconduct With Students; Soccer Mom Wanted On 10 Accounts Of Sex With Minors.*

No wonder people have begun to feel it is safer to keep their hands to themselves at all times.

At the same time however, legitimate massage therapists and dubious massage "parlors" are jammed with clients. All craving the same things... human physical contact. Clearly, we are a touch-starved culture.

All of us, however, have a need to touch and be touched. This innate need is know as the healing touch and has been a part of medicine for thousands of years, but medicine has become so scientific that the art of medicine is struggling to keep from being buried under technology.

Dr. Mehmet Oz at Presbyterian Hospital in New York coined a new term, Global Medicine. He states, "Global Medicine refers to the idea that in little more than a decade, linkages between health care technologies of different cultures and continents have merged, resulting in global medicine technology. The next generation of young scientists and clinicians from both the research and clinical communities are merging established ancient technologies (like touch therapy) from outside the U.S. with modern medical technology and forging new ground in an increasingly challenging health care climate."

In a research paper entitled, "Haptic Medicine" written by Cindy Mason, CMT, PhD, a research associate at Stanford University in Palo Alto, Ca. and founder of Humans Without Boarders, she shares multiple research studies done on the positive medical effects of touch for everything from Aggression, Alzheimer's, and Asthma to blood flow and blood pressure issues, to Cancer, Chronic Fatigue Syndrome, and Cognition (Learning) to Diabetes to Organ Transplants to Spinal Cord Injuries and even Stroke, and several other conditions. One interesting case study she reports on has to do with a set of twin girls born at Stanford University Medical Center in May 1995. The twins were born prematurely and the smaller of the two was not doing well. In fact she was not expected to live. They were placed in their respective incubators. A nurse decided to fight hospital policy and put the twins in one incubator together, lying them side by side. Immediately the larger, healthier twin placed her arm over the back of her sister and kept it there. Shortly, the smaller twin's heart rate stabilized, her body temperature normalized and from then on began to thrive. This is a great example of that innate need to touch and be touched demonstrated by humans to young to be taught this belief.

48

All of us, however, have a need to touch and be touched. Others of us *thrive* on human touch. When I look back over my life, the loneliest, most challenging times where when I was receiving the least amount of human touch. As a young mother I blossomed while holding and cuddling my boys. I wore a pouch and carried them on me almost all the time. Many people said I was spoiling them, but in reality I think I was spoiling myself.

We All Need Touch -- However....

I've traveled around the world a bit and come to realize that we Americans tend to touch very little compared to many other countries. Research shows that two Americans setting in a restaurant will touch on the average of twice in an hour. When compared to the French who touch on an average of 110 times in that same time period and the Puerto Ricans who touch 180 times, we Americans are a culture of touch starved people.

Phyllis K. Davis wrote a book titled, "The Power Of Touch" where she reports on her own and other's studies of why we deprive ourselves of this incredibly important gift when it is at our "fingertips". She states three reasons. One, there is a misconception that people who touch frequently are promiscuous. Second, there is the fear of being labeled as homosexual. And third, the Freudian concept has managed to prevail, even in our educated society today, that children will develop sexual feelings for their parents if they are touched too much.

I can't say whether I agree with her beliefs or not, but I have witnessed personally that parents tend to decrease the amount of touching with their children as they reach puberty.

But I feel it is a combination of the social pressure on both the child and the parent. Why do so many fathers and sons feel it is only acceptable to hug or high-five if the son hits a home run or scores a touch down?

I found it challenging as my boys became older and started shunning my hugs or touch, especially when in public. It just wasn't socially acceptable to be touched by your mother after a certain age. It said, "He's a mommy's boy" and their friends would make fun of them. This saddened me a great deal. Young boys and mothers need that continuation of casual contact.

When one of my son's was playing Little League baseball I got talked into coaching his team. Honestly, it didn't take too much convincing, except that I was the first and only female coach in our town. So I expected a few doubtful looks from dads. (But then, they hadn't volunteered to coach....) What I didn't expect, in the wild atmosphere of coaching little leaguers was to learn a lesson about the social view of touching.

One evening, in the middle of a game, I had turned third-base coaching over to a high school player who was helping me. I was leaning against the fence watching the game, making mental notes of what skills I'd need to address in our next practice and talking to one of the other fathers who was coaching a rival team. During the next at-bat, one of my team members made it to third base.

I stepped away from the fence, telling the other coach I'd be right back. I called time out and stepped over to the boy on my team, knelt down and tied his shoe laces. Then I stood, removed his hat, tousled his hair, and told him he was doing great – "But you need to keep your shoes tied, buddy." Then I nodded to the umpire to continue the game, and returned to the fence.

When I got back to the fence, the other coach was laughing and shaking his head at me. "What?" I asked, really not understanding. My actions were just so natural, I hadn't really even thought about what I was doing.

He said, "You know, none of us fathers could ever get away with doing something that nurturing. We would be laughed at. And if we were too free in making physical contact with their kids, parents would be screaming to get someone else to coach their boys. I don't touch anyone."

I thought how sad it was that he felt that guarded, and also that perhaps he was right. We don't allow for healthy nurturing touch in public, especially between boys and men.

I imagine my sensitivity to touch is one of the reasons I was intuitively drawn to this work. Because so much of what I do is communicated with my hands I have learned to palpate even the slightest variance in tissues, breathing and emotions being transferred through the body and into my hands.

Robert Fulford, DO, said that when he was training with Dr. Sutherland they would put a strand of human hair underneath a sheet of paper and practice refining their sense of touch to the point that they could trace that strand of hair. Once they mastered that, they placed a second sheet of paper on top of the hair, and then a third. Feeling a piece of hair under sheets of paper is not an easy task, but by practicing this technique the practitioner can develop an amazing skill of palpitation.

Another way to enhance this touch is to train with your eyes closed. We are all aware of how a person who has lost or was born without one of their **sensory functions** will experience a greater degree of sensitivity in their remaining senses. The same thing often happens when you watch someone who is thoroughly enjoying some food they have just taken a bite of; they momentarily close their eyes instinctively savoring the enhancement of their sense of taste. Or have you ever watched someone who loves music when they are listening to a favorite piano sonata? They too will often shut their eyes and sometimes as they do this, their fingers will begin to move. The sense of hearing is being heightened and the pure joy brought on by that sense is communicating unconsciously to their hands to move.

When I am working with someone and trying to read their body, I will close my eyes and settle my senses into my palms and my fingers. Often, if the client and I have been speaking, I will slow my responses to their comments, both in the cadence of my words and also the time between sentences. This is a conscious move on my part to the unconscious part of their brain that it is now time to quiet down and listen with their body. As this happens, the client will almost always grow quiet and I can now take away both sight and sound and focus on the communication that is occurring solely through touch.

I'd like to try and demystify how touch heals the patient's body as best I can in the following chapters. We've talked about the pulses and that it is the rhythm of these pulses that are dictating my touch but sometimes the work becomes as much intuitive as it does physical. By this I mean that there are cases where the body does not follow the path of revealing what it needs or responds as the "textbook" says it should. This is when I call on a higher power to help me. I speak about this specifically in one of the case studies and will get into it in more detail at that time. You may initially want to label this notion as religious, and not wanting to get involved in any particular form of healing that has to do with a religious or spiritual nature, shun it without further exploration. But doesn't all healing, whether traditional Western medicine or the alternative Eastern medicines have some form of spirituality involved in them? Perhaps it isn't spoken of frequently, but, if you asked most doctors, they would tell you of times they have been at a loss of what to do and when they were quiet and meditative they remembered some obscure case study in an article or text book that gave them insight, or when they prayed for guidance because they were at a loss of what to do next, an idea came to them. Medical doctors are known to act on hunches or intuition. This is the spiritual side of healing. It is where known or remembered logic ends and the gut takes over. It occurs in medicine and it occurs in Craniosacral Therapy.

Now that we've discussed the merits of Western Medicine, the role of Complimentary Medicine, the history and theory of Craniosacral Therapy and the path to wellness, as well as the importance of touch, I would like to introduce you to a few of my clients and their experiences with CST and the complimentary adjunct therapies I use in my office.

Chapter 5

The Head Is Foundational

Ricky

The first time Ricky came to my office, he marched in, a large boy for his tender age of 6. When he saw me, a stranger to him, he hesitated, the uncertainty written on his face. "Where's Mmmmmrs. Sssstenson?" he asked his mother as he drew in close to her. "Whossssse sssssshe?"

"Ricky, this is Annette, she's going to help you learn to talk better like Mrs. Stenson, but she is going to do it in a little different way," his mother said as she reassuringly put her arm around his shoulders. Ricky didn't look convinced.

When his mother had originally called me on the telephone to schedule this appointment she had shared Ricky's story. He was slow developing speech. When he did finally start speaking it was very difficult to understand him, which was then followed by stuttering. The family noticed the condition became worse when he was fatigued or under stress. They had taken him first to their pediatrician who then referred him to an Ear Nose and Throat specialist. He found nothing unusual so had arranged for hearing tests. Those also came back normal. He was then referred to a neurologist to see if there was brain involvement.

It was then that Ricky was diagnosed with Developmental Dysphasia which is an inability to pronounce words or poor enunciation, not due to muscle weakness, but due to lack of ability to convey the thought from the brain to the mouth; causing difficulty in developing expressive language skills. In short, Ricky knew what he wanted to say, but just couldn't get his mouth to cooperate.

He had been in speech therapy through the school district shortly after his diagnoses at age four. They made minor advances but nothing significant. Now almost 7 years old and in second grade a new set of problems were emerging. His school work was suffering, he was being disruptive in class, showing common symptoms of Attention Deficit Disorder, and getting into fights with other classmates. The other children were teasing him because of the way he talked, and this was taking a blow to his young self esteem. However, due to his size he soon realized that physical force quieted the taunts and teasing. It also meant spending more and more time in "time out" or in the Principal's office.

Ricky was quickly developing the dreaded label as "The Problem Student". His frightened and frustrated parent's wanted to change the path he was headed down, and have him "just become the sweet contented boy they used to have".

When working with children, I've found it is important to put them at ease as quickly as possible. This is often done by letting them bring and hold a small toy or book. Many therapists find this disruptive or distracting; however, I find the child's emotional comfort to be the most important part of the appointment. If the child is happy, they hold still better, and they are more cooperative when I need them to talk to me or do something for me.

In Ricky's case he had brought a DVD player with a favorite movie. His mother was concerned that he would still not lie down because he had a rough day at school and was very restless. I told Ricky his mother was going to wait in the other room. He could watch the movie and when we were done we would have his mother come back in. I don't always ask parents to leave, but when a parent is as apprehensive as she was, it spills over to the child. I suggested she check in with us in about 10 minutes. She said to call her if he didn't cooperate.

When I cradled Ricky's head to observe his cranial rhythm I waited, and waited. The first notable observation was he had no cranial rhythm. So I moved to the lower back/sacral junction to observe it there. Here I was able to detect a slow, shallow rhythm. Beginning here I followed the rhythm and then nudged it further into both extension and flexion hoping to enhance the flow enough that it would engage the cranial bones. The tissues softened, loosening tension and allowing the rhythm to flow more freely.

I returned again to Ricky's head hoping the rhythm would now be present there. There was still nothing happening. So systematically I began to release each of the cranial bones, starting with the frontal bone. As I began to gently nudge this bone into flexion and extension it was as if I could see a zigzag line going from the center of the frontal bone through the middle of his skull to the back of the head. This is the midline of the head where the Falx cerebri membrane separates the two hemispheres of the brain containing the parietal lobes. This membrane attaches to the frontal bone. When this membrane is tight it will pull the frontal bone tight against the frontal lobe of the brain creating a slight pressure or compression on the brain.

It is important to note here that the frontal lobe of the brain controls the expression of language and the parietal lobes controls the understanding of language.

As I gently tried to lift the frontal bone away from the brain and straight up to stretch the membrane and try to "straighten it out" from its strange pattern Ricky gave an audible sigh. His eyelids fluttered and within seconds he was sound asleep. It was as though his brain finally took a breath, felt such relief from the years of compression and immediately relaxed. Then it was as if watching a wave gently roll over Ricky's body as his shoulders relaxed onto the table, his breath deepened, his arms fell open at his sides and his legs relaxed rolling out so his feet splayed open, allowing his body to totally relax. When I could finally feel a significant flexion and extension of the frontal bone I moved on to the parietal bones. This is done by very gently and with consistent pressure pulling the hair away from the roots. At first there wasn't any give and Ricky began to stir as though disturbed, but within about one minute the bones began to lift and stretch the sutures holding the bones compressed too tightly together. Again he sighed and fully reverted back to the fully relaxed position. At this point I was beginning to wonder how difficult a birthing experience Ricky's mother had with him. This type of severe compression of skull bones in a child is often indicative of prolonged labor or a difficult delivery.

His mother poked her head into the room, surprised that she hadn't heard anything from her son or me through the open doorway. Imagine her surprise when she found her overly active, non-attentive, no nap for years, son lying sound asleep on my table.

After releasing the remaining cranial bones to make sure they were moving in synchrony with the frontal and parietal bones I moved to the ears. There should be a slight give and then a feeling as though fresh soft taffy were being pulled. Ricky's ears were as rigid as his skull had been when I started the treatment. By gently pulling on the ear lobes I can instigate a stretching of the Tentorium membrane which separates the temporal lobes of the brain. Stretching this membrane releases tension on these lobes. This is critical as the temporal lobe controls behavior. This is critical when it comes to treating Attention Deficit Disorder or Hyperactivity or even Autism.

Ricky's mother reported that he slept all the way home, awakened long enough to eat some dinner and then went to bed and slept nearly 12 hours. This is indicative of a central nervous system that has been working massive overtime for a long period of time.

I saw Ricky three additional times each time stretching the membranes to assure optimum brain function. However, on his second visit, using the cranial rhythm to access what else was happening in his body, I discovered that he needed mouth work. This can be somewhat difficult with a child, especially one who tends to fall asleep on the table because they can't keep their mouth open and will bite me. So I needed to engage Ricky in conversation with yes/no answers. I told him I would ask him questions and he was to hold up one finger for yes and two fingers for no. It's a game so most children will buy into it at least for a short period of time.

What I discovered with Ricky was that the roof of his mouth was locked and not moving into the flexion/extension movement. Also his vomer bone, which is a small but important bone that helps form the nasal septum, was jammed upward too high.

After making adjustments on these bones I asked his mother if he had sucked his thumb as a baby or young child. She indicated he had. A child who sucks their thumb almost always has a stuck vomer or maxilla (roof of the mouth). The sucking motion temporarily reduces the pressure these misaligned bones are causing in the cranium, which brings relief and comfort to the child.

After Ricky's first appointment the teachers, speech therapist and all family members started to see changes in Ricky. He was much calmer, slept easily and soundly, was able to concentrate when given a task, and a minor improvement was noted in his speech. However, after the second visit, a week later, when the mouth work was completed a second time and the membranes stretched again, Ricky made significant headway. His progress was remarkable on a daily basis. His speech therapist was astounded to see the difference two weeks had made compared to the almost three years she had spent in therapy with Ricky.

After four weekly visits we moved Ricky's appointments to half hour monthly sessions until school was out. After that I felt we had reached the point of maximum help I could give him. His speech was almost normal and the stutter was gone. His parents and teachers reported that stress and fatigue still triggered slips backward. So at this point it became necessary to also look at lifestyle and behavior patterns in the family which we will discuss later in chapter 12.

Studies done by Viola Frymann, DO and the Osteopathic Center for Children & Families in San Diego, have demonstrated that children with compression to the delicate bones that make up the infant skull can result in neurological dysfunction such as Attention Deficit Disorder, sensory development and autism. As the baby descends into the mother's pelvis during birth, the pubic bone can exert pressure on parts of the skull. This can cause stress on the tissue resulting in strain patterns. Using instruments such as forceps or vacuum extraction can further put the baby at risk for cranial bone dysfunction. It is important to recognize, however, that such instrumentation may be a life-saving measure and should be used if deemed necessary. However, if these babies could be evaluated and treated by an osteopath or cranial therapist as soon after birth as possible, the long term effects would be minimized.

Research has found that these strains can alter the soft tissue underneath the skull which can change blood flow patterns to the brain itself. Gentle manipulation by a therapist trained in cranial osteopathy or craniosacral therapy can significantly improve the symptoms in these children. In a 3-year study of 286 children, Dr. Frymann demonstrated that osteopathic treatment improved sensory, intellectual, and motor performance in children with neurological problems. Research conducted at Michigan State University further corroborated Dr. Frymann's findings.

Steve

I was at a social gathering of the local triathlon group of which I was a member of when a 6' tall, lean young man approached me. He introduced himself as Steve and asked if he could get some professional advice. He indicated that he had been athletic ever since junior high school, playing all sports through high school. During his college years he had started cycling and had enjoyed that for several years now. Three years ago at the age of 30 he had joined this group and started training for triathlons. He had progressively improved as he became proficient in swimming and revisited his cross country days of running. However, in the past few months he found his lower back and groin hurt and his calf would cramp severely causing him to shorten his workouts or have to skip them altogether. "I'm too young to feel this bad," he said trying to joke about it but I could hear the desperation in his voice. It was true; he was too young to be experiencing that kind of pain.

I suggested he make an appointment so we could try to unwind the tissues and figure out what was going on. He had never had any massage or body work but he had previously had a few chiropractic adjustments which helped for a day or two, but the pain and cramping always returned. I assured him that it was probably either muscular and/or physiological and that I could help with that. He committed to three appointments and to suspend workouts for two weeks.

When Steve arrived at my office I noticed that he walked heavier on the left side favoring ever so slightly the right side of his body. On physical inspection I noted that his right hip was a good inch and a half higher than his left and rotated marginally posterior (towards his back). This would account for the strain on the groin muscle on that side as the tissues were constantly being stretched upwards and pulled backward. As I told Steve this, he said, "Yes, that is what the chiropractor had adjusted both times." It seemed fairly simple that his back and hip flexor muscles were out of balance causing a torque in the pelvis.

As I cradled Steve's head and monitored the cranial rhythm it was adequate with some obvious compression at the base of the skull. When I went to the lower back/sacral area to monitor it from this location there was very little rhythm and his lower back was rigid. Even toned muscles have a suppleness about them but his lower back was more like a plank of wood than supple toned muscles. So I guided the cranial rhythm into the direction of ease, or the direction it was moving the greatest, and then held it, monitoring the texture of the tissues. Shortly the fascia began to unwind. As it begins to move I simply follow it, not letting it turn back or pull back into where it had been. It is similar to trying to untie knots in a string, twisting it this way and that to get the string to lie flat and straight. There is a muscle on each side of the back that starts at the last rib and goes down and connects into the hip bone called the QL (quadratus lumborum). When one or both of these muscles are tight or slack they play havoc with the pelvis being aligned. This was the case with Steve. His QLs were in spasm. Once the fascia of these mirrored muscles finished unwinding they were much more in the normal limits of tension.

So at this point I moved to the front of the pelvis in the groin area and palpated the hip flexor muscles which help us bend at the waist, as well as lift our legs as we walk, climb, run or cycle. Again his muscles were very rigid and also painful if I used too much pressure. The left was tighter than the right, causing the pull down of the left hip and the heavier stride on that side of his body. I used the same myofascial release I had on his QLs, but with lighter pressure due to the sensitivity of the muscles and also of the groin area in general.

As I began to release particularly the left side, his left calf began to cramp just like in his workout. This indicated to me that the fascial restrictions he was experiencing in his groin were extending down the leg and either squeezing the calf muscles or torque them making them cramp. I followed the path of the fascia down the outside of the left thigh and as I approached the knee area the cramping abruptly stopped. When I checked the calf muscles they were supple and normal indicating they were a response to the problem in the groin and leg, not a true symptom.

I worked on Steve's neck and the base of his skull to help keep the cranial rhythm moving at the healthy rate it was now producing. But I felt the majority of Steve's symptoms came from the lower back and groin. So when he returned four days later saying that he had felt great for two days and then slowly the stiffness and pain had returned and that today he was hurting, I was surprised. The calves had not cramped again, but still I had expected more relief than this.

The second appointment was much like the first, but I was able to go a little deeper into the groin abdominal area. Steve assured me he had never had any type of abdominal surgery to complicate things so I continued on the premise of muscle strain, and muscle spasms causing an imbalance of the pelvic structure. He felt great when he left. We scheduled him to return in 5 days. To my surprise he called on day four and said he was really hurting in his left hip and could hardly walk. When he arrived at the office I could see the discouragement and pain on his grim face and in his slumped posture. His body language of rounded shoulders, slow deliberate steps and dull eyes belied his pain and a desire to give up.

I knew I was missing something so I sat down with Steve and reviewed his health history form. He had indicated that he did not have any jaw/TMJ pain and that he had not had anything more than regular dental cleanings in the past year. No surgeries or scars to deal with. I was rather stumped so I turned to his body for direction. I cradled his head and waited. The rhythm was adequate but certainly not what it was when he had left the two previous appointments. I settled in, closed my eyes and focused on what information would come through my hands. It took a while before I noticed a slight pull to the right in the beginning and the end of the rhythm cycle. Asking the body to use it's rhythm, I asked if the lesion was structural, visceral,(organ) or emotional.   The rhythm stopped abruptly when I said structural indicating a *yes* that this was primarily a structural issue. Because the tension pull in the cranial system was at my finger tips and just beyond, I assumed the lesion was in the cranium, but I asked to make sure. The body indicated yes again by the CSR stopping.   I systematically went through the bones of the head. Each came up negative for misalignment. I asked the rhythm if it was in his mouth and bam I got a resounding yes. The CSR which had been moving steadily just stopped abruptly. I again verbally asked Steve about dental work. He said, "No, nothing had been done." But then he said about a year and a half ago he had a tooth crack and they had put a crown on it on the upper right side. Sure enough when I went in his mouth the roof of his mouth was compressed upward pressing on the sinus area. He had only minor flexion and extension on the right side of the roof of his mouth which was gradually shutting down his entire rhythm after I would get it going.

The hip joints and the jaw joints will always compensate for each other. They are the two largest joints on each end of the spine. The body wants to keep our spine straight more than it wants to keep hips or jaw joints level. So if the jaw slips out of alignment due to injury, having the jaw propped open for long periods of time, or misalignment of the way the teeth come together, the hips will shift to compensate and keep the spine aligned. In Steve's case the new crown he had placed was just a touch higher than his natural teeth. (It only takes the thickness of a hair.) Therefore when he wasn't thinking about it, probably when sleeping, he would grind his teeth around trying to find a comfortable position for the jaw. He found one, but it was not an optimal functioning one so other bones and muscles adapted. Over time his hip needed to adjust and compensate which caused undue stress on the hip flexors. As they shifted and pulled the hip slightly the QLs tried to adjust, but finally started yelling with pain.

Once we made the corrections in the mouth and Steve went back to his dentist to have the crown adjusted, he then held his adjustments with me and we were able to make progress in retraining the jaw/neck muscles to relax as well as the lower back, groin and hip flexors.

We also started adding rehabilitative exercises that taught the body how to use specific muscles properly now that they were supple and mobile. This is critical so that the muscles and the bones they support learn to act in balance again. We also added routine ice baths after difficult workouts to help release the lactic acid build-up and decrease inflammation.

These types of compensations don't happen overnight. It takes months and sometimes years of slow adaptation. We eventually had to add a magnesium citrate (a natural muscle relaxant) supplement to Steve's diet to help his muscles relax when he wasn't working them in his training. But with the jaw work, the muscle work, the new exercises and the ice baths he was able to complete his next triathlon without undue pain or stress to his body.

Chapter 6

It May Not Be What You Think It Is

In the previous chapter I introduced you to Steve, whose lower back (and eventually knee/leg) problems were not exactly what other practitioners had thought it was. Usually, when we have recurring or chronic pain in one area of the body we think there is something wrong *in that area*. Over and over during my years of treating clients, however, I have found that the issue in one area is a result of dysfunction in some other area of the body; or it is being intensified because the person is compensating in other parts of the body... sometimes even in other areas of their life.

Ben

Consider Ben, who I mentioned earlier. Ben was a 50-year-old male, working for a technology company on an executive level. His job carried with it a great deal of daily stress. He suffered from severe headaches that presented very much like migraines. Ben's headache would begin as an overwhelming fatigue, followed by a low-grade tension at the base of his skull. The tension would continue to build and then spread to cover most of the left side of his head. His eye on the left would begin to throb, then tear and swell.

As with most migraines, the pain would last three days no matter what Ben did to try and get rid of it. He was taking pain medication which helped him cope, but after a day and a half of that he would find himself too nauseated to keep the medication down.

One clue that tipped me off from the start that the root of Ben's problem laid elsewhere was that the traditional medications for migraines, such as Imitrex, didn't help Ben. He'd also undergone both a CT scan and an MRI which showed everything to be normal. During the new client interview I noted that stress both at work and at home were high. Even though Ben's diet wasn't what I like to see, he reported that he had tried tracking the headaches to foods and hadn't found any connection. What he'd eaten before one headache he could eat at another time with no resulting headache. I noted on physical exam that his right hip was about an inch higher than the left and that he stood with a slight shift to the left. His left shoulder was higher than the right and also more rounded forward. The left ear was slightly higher than the right one.

These structural patterns reinforced the suspicion that these headaches were probably muscle tension headaches causing an inflammation of the trigeminal nerve, or what's known as Trigeminal Neuralgia. The pattern of pain he was describing fit the pathway of the nerve. When the muscles got out of balance and tense they would spasm causing contraction and squeezing on the nerve. When a nerve is compressed by its surrounding muscles it will become inflamed, which causes severe pain.

In Ben's case this caused a severe headache. In others, however, depending on what nerves are being compressed, it can cause pain in the shoulders or even radiating pain down the arms. A person can have wrist and hand pain and numb fingers (which is often thought to be Carpel Tunnel Syndrome), when in fact the muscles in the neck are so tight they are causing a compression on the Median Nerve that exits the spine in the lower part of the neck where it attaches to the shoulders.

Nadia

Nadia, a 38 year old personal assistant to the CEO of a major IT company came to me saying she had been diagnosed with Carpel Tunnel from repetitive use of her computer key board and that she had undergone the recommended surgery and physical therapy – only to find that she still had numbness in her fingers and her hands hurt all the time. Sadly, no one had bothered looking at her neck or the way her teeth came together and the instability the bite was creating in her cervical vertebrae. Yet when I examined her neck she had limited mobility turning right or left. There was also major decrease of movement when leaning her head backward indicating compression at the base of the skull.

I asked, "Are you aware of clenching or grinding your teeth."

"I don't think so. Not that I'm aware of," she replied.

I clarified. "When you're sitting at the computer, or watching TV, or driving, do your teeth touch? Are they touching now?" Most people don't realize that, normally, your teeth should never touch except when chewing or swallowing.

"Oh. Yeah. They're touching," she indicated.

I knew that her jaws were clenching – a common sign of compression at the base of the skull.

This is a connection most people do not know, including many healthcare professionals: The way your jaws and teeth come together have a significant impact on the body's overall structure. For instance in Nadia's case she was constantly clenching her teeth which caused a contraction and eventual shortening of the muscles used for chewing. As these muscles shortened they forced the lower jaw to move backward toward the ear decreasing joint space in the jaw joint itself. This displacement of the lower jaw and muscle spasming causes tension in the trapezius muscle that runs from the base of the skull to the clavicle bone in the front of the body and the shoulder blades on the back of the body. If this tightness is left untreated it will eventually result in a rounding of the shoulders as the body tries to ease some of the tension of the trapezius muscle causing the shoulders to rise upward toward the ears. Since the trapezius muscle overlays the muscles that support the cervical spine (the neck), as it contracts it causes a compression of the vertebrae in the spine underneath it. This compacted vertebrae then puts pressure on the nerves that exit the spine around them causing pain somewhere along the path of the nerve, which is often times the end point, which is the wrist and hand.

As I noted at the outset of this chapter, our problems can radiate from parts of the body we would not associate with the site of the pain.

Daniel

When Daniel, a 42 year old male who worked as a sales representative for a golfing company came in to my office he was complaining of pain in his right shoulder. He could barely turn his head to the left to look over his shoulder which was making driving difficult and dangerous. He spent much of his day driving from one golf pro shop or golf course to another. He told me this pain and stiffness had been going on for several weeks. It would get really bad for a couple of days and then seem to get a little better for several days and then flare up again. He had received a deep tissue massage with the focus on the upper back, shoulders and neck. It had helped for a couple of days. He had also gone to his chiropractor twice and had his neck adjusted. That had helped for two days each time, but the pain would return. During his new client interview I noted that he loved his job and felt very little stress associated with it. However, just spending so much time driving in heavy traffic each day did tend to wear him down. He reported at the end of the day he really enjoyed a nice glass of wine to help his body relax.

Upon physical evaluation the tension in his upper back and shoulders was noteworthy. It was as if he had a board in there instead of nice supple strong muscles. His hips were level but the right one was rotated slightly forward of the left. There seemed to be a twisting of his body forward from the right side. This would in turn cause a pulling on the muscles on the left side of his body, including the neck, decreasing his flexibility and range of motion. Without clearing the twisting pattern in the pelvis all the way up the back, all the shoulder/neck work in town would not have cleared up his pain.

In order to get resolution to the pain and lack of function they were experiencing, with each of these clients, I needed to look at the entire body, from the mouth, to the base of the skull to the tail bone and everything in between. I can't emphasize enough that many times the issue isn't what the client thinks it is.

For Daniel, I had to adjust his bite by releasing the muscles and soft tissues inside the mouth as well as have him wear a dental appliance that would help open his bite a small amount. This is sometimes necessary in order to lengthen the muscles back to their natural length after they've shortened from extended contraction. The mouth work was completed using a number of craniosacral techniques. I also did craniosacral therapy to open the base of the skull by releasing the soft tissue in that area to keep compression off the cranial nerves as they exit the skull. Doing a sacral (tailbone) decompression helped to alleviate the tension in the pelvis causing his hips to misalign. I don't know which came first the misalignment of the hips or the bite, but obviously they were playing off each other and causing severe fascial torsion patterns along the spine. This is what I call the "teeter/totter" effect. You can fix one end but it will just move to the other end of the spine and when that end acts in response you will be right back where you started. The bite and the hips must be fixed simultaneously.

With Nadia, it was much the same story except hers was almost all head, neck and shoulder, including mouth work that needed unwinding and relaxing so the nerve compression could be eliminated. However, because the nerve had been compressed for some time, it took several weeks after achieving the decompression for the nerve to calm down and all the pain resolve out of her hands and wrists. Even though all her pain was in the wrists and hands, I only worked in that area once after treating the core issue of the pain.

Daniel required four appointments spent mostly doing fascial release and craniosacral balancing of the soft tissues in his pelvis, trunk of the body and his neck. Once we got the layers of twisting fascia straightened out he was able to turn his head nearly 90 degrees both right and left and the pain in the right shoulder left without returning.

In Conclusion

In my experience, the reason most people's pain is not relieved stems from the fact that many practitioners only focus on the area of concern rather than on the patient's whole body. Even when a physician sends a patient to a physical therapist, usually they will ask the therapist to work on an arm, a leg, a neck, or whatever part of the body is hurting. But because the core issue is often overlooked, which could be at the other end of the body, the pain returns or the injury reoccurs.

For this reason whole body therapy is critical. This is why you will need to find a therapist who honors the body as a whole entity and will exam and work with the entire body. Also as you have seen in the previous chapter's case studies, as well as, the ones mentioned here, neither you nor your practitioner can rely on your symptoms or conscious thought process to relieve your pain or dysfunction. As I stated previously the practitioner and yourself must rely on your body's inner self to reveal what it needs and proceed from there.

Chapter 7

PTSD (Post Traumatic Stress Disorder) and Cranial Work

You will recall back in chapter two I talked about Emotional Release Therapy as one of the adjunct therapies I use with craniosacral therapy. Often a client will arrive with what seems like a standard physical issue, like high blood pressure, or insomnia or persistent pain in a specific area. However, when I start working on this person the regular techniques I use to release the tissues don't work or they work, but, the same tissue area is right back to where we started when they return on subsequent visits. This is an indication that there is another, deeper cause for the issue at hand. Often there are strong emotional component involved.

Releasing these powerful emotional feelings from the tissues can improve symptoms significantly for those experiencing Post Traumatic Stress Disorder as well as all other emotionally based disorders such as depression, anxiety, and hyper-vigilance, or hyper-sensitive disorders. The case study I'm sharing with you today is based on a military associated PTSD, however, PTSD can be experienced by anyone who has gone through a severe traumatic situation in their life.

Aaron

Aaron, a 53 year old retired Army colonel who had spent his last several years of service on the Hostage Rescue Team, came to see me with complaints of not being able to sleep, nightmares, and occasionally tightness of breath. He said his wife and children said he had changed and was often more irritable and short tempered with them. He also suffered occasional headaches but other than that was in excellent health and physical condition with a body fat of a lean 10%.

He felt he was managing fine taking Ambien as needed for his insomnia and Zoloft for his anxieties. If his headaches got too bad he had a prescription for a non-narcotic drug, Tramadol.

He was currently a partner in a high tech security company with a government contract developing, maintaining, and training military personnel to use the devices or technology their firm developed. Aaron reported that his job could be stressful, "at times, like when deadlines where looming". Or "when we aren't finished with the development of a device and the funds are running out for that specific project."

I asked him about personal relationships at home, friends, and co-workers. He said all was fine except his family's concern about him being irritable. When I asked him if he agreed with their assessment he replied, "Maybe a little when I'm under stress at work."

Aaron's wife had done research on the internet and wondered if he didn't suffer from a mild case of Post-Traumatic Stress Syndrome (PTSD). She had also read where craniosacral therapy helped PTSD sufferers and wanted him to try a few sessions. When Aaron explained this, I asked again if he agreed with her assessment. His body became more rigid, sitting up straight and tall, squaring his shoulders and gave an almost imperceptible shrug. I waited another few seconds or so and when he didn't respond any further or break eye contact I knew I wasn't going to get much more of an answer from him. I explained how the body holds onto memories of events when the person feels strong emotions. "I would expect in the type of work you did while with the Army, you experienced some intense times where you felt strong emotions." (Review chapter two, pages 30-31 for further explanation)

My first observation as I'd just observed in our interview, he did not want to discuss emotions. His face remained flat and unreadable of emotion when I brought up what he'd seen in combat.

Second, there was his physical demeanor. Aaron, was still sitting tall and rigid, almost as if at attention, when he finally responded, "You have no idea what I have seen or experienced. We didn't get emotional about it. We just did our duty."

I had observed Aaron walking as I followed him down the hall and into the treatment room. His gait was evenly balanced, hips level, shoulders level. His posture seemed in good shape. However, he moved very quickly, almost precisely, not at all the calm relaxed walk of most people, even if they are a little nervous about their first session with me.

75

The third observation was Aaron's speech pattern. It was also rapid, nearly staccato. I wasn't sure if this was normal for him or if he felt he had other things to accomplish and didn't really want to take the time to be here.

The Hands On Session

We began with Aaron laying face up on the table, lights low and soft music. Like everyone receiving craniosacral therapy he remained fully clothed but with the top button of his shirt opened, tie off, and shirt sleeves unbuttoned creating a more relaxing atmosphere. I suggested he try to relax and let go for the next several minutes. He chuckled a little sarcastically and said, "Yeah, like that's going to happen. I have fifty things on my mind, and relaxing isn't one of them."

 This is the response of many adults I work on. I don't argue or try to persuade them otherwise. I know that most people when not challenged will fall asleep or at least dose off and on during the treatment. However, people who suffer from anxiety disorders, such as PTSD, exacerbated by physical trauma will need a couple of appointments before their nervous systems will "let go" enough to let them fall asleep. Such was the case with Aaron. It would take several sessions before he could let down the protective barrier he'd built around him, like an invisible "armor."

It is important to note that when working with someone who requires emotional release work, like Aaron would, I want to achieve a state of relaxation for him. However, when doing the actual emotional release work I need to keep them in the present moment. With military personnel like Aaron, giving them a direct assignment, such as breathe in for 5 counts, hold for 2, and release the breath for 5 counts will often work well. These people are used to being given an assignment or taking and giving orders so the therapist needs to be firm and direct with them. However, with someone whose trauma involved an experience were their will was taken from them, held hostage, rape, etc, the therapist needs to engage the client to keep them present by asking them specific questions, such as, "What color of blouse do I have on?", "How many pictures are on the walls in this room?", The trick is to have the client revisit the experience, identify the emotion(s), and give permission to release the emotion without losing the client to the experience itself.

During Aaron's first appointment I released several physical blockages, such as tension in and around his shoulder blades and neck extending to the base of his skull which was slowing down the CSR. Occasionally, I would ask Aaron if he could feel the heat emanating from under my hand, which indicates a release of the tissues. Each time he said no. I was not surprised, because when people have experienced trauma one of the first things they do is disassociate with their physical bodies so they don't have to feel anything that might remind them of the trauma. I didn't push this acknowledgement, yet. This first appointment needed to be about building trust because instinctively I knew Aaron and I would be visiting some pretty ugly places and events if he stuck with me.

At the end of that first appointment he admitted he felt more relaxed than he could ever remember. I asked him to commit to coming three more times in one week intervals. I explained that it is important to make that commitment and stick to it if we were going to make progress. If too much time (much more than a week) goes by between visits it is almost like starting over again, rather than building on the previous appointment. He agreed and we set his appointment for one week.

Connecting With Himself

As Aaron approached the treatment room I again noticed his quick stride. He always looks like he is in a hurry, I thought to myself. I asked what he had noticed different since our last visit. He paused, thought for a minute, and said, "nothing really."

I asked how he had slept the night of his appointment.

"Oh yes, I did sleep good that night. In fact I was kind of wiped out all that evening." Good, we had made a crack in the armor. He took off his tie, loosened his collar and shirt sleeves and lay down on the table. I had to smile to myself. It was as if he were saying, "No time for small talk. Let's get this done."

As I cradled Aaron's head and sat observing his CSR and listening to his body, he said, "Wow! Your hands are really warm today. Are you feeling ok?"

I smiled! "That's your body, not mine."

"No way!"

For the first time in a very long time, Aaron was noticing a subtle nudge from within his body. That was a great start. I was then directed to his lower back and placed my hands there. I began to initiate a fascial release of the area but the tissues didn't respond. I could tell from the heat and tension coming from the area, and the lack of physical response of the tissues that we needed to release the emotions held in this area.

I approached this next part of the appointment with a little dread. Emotional release work is very different from what most people expect when they come for "bodywork". Most of the time a client has never experienced someone "reading" their body. They are shocked to have someone know information about them that they have often times suppressed and not discussed with anyone in a long time, or perhaps never discussed. It is a totally new approach for them to have me address their emotions when they are coming to me for physical issues.

Let's briefly review again what we discussed back in chapter two about the emotional release technique. I am using the craniosacral rhythm (the CSR) as my indicator. As I cradle a part of the body with my hands and ask the body questions, I observe the CSR. When the answer to the question is "yes", the rhythm will stop and when the answer is "no" the rhythm speeds up. The patient's rhythm and my hands tell the story.

Back to Aaron's story. I began to monitor Aaron's CSR, asking for a positive or yes indication, the rhythm stopped. I then asked the body for a negative or no indication and the rhythm sped up. Now that I had my indicator I could begin to ask the body via the CSR pertinent questions of Aaron's body.

"When did you first feel the emotion that is locked here? Zero to 5 years, 5 – 10, 10-15?" The rhythm stopped. "10, 11, 12" and the rhythm stopped.

"Was it the first half or the year ?" No. "Second half of the year?" Yes.

"Did it have to do with another person?" Yes.

"Was it male?" Yes.

"Did it have to do with work?" Yes.

"What emotion is being held here? Anger, fear," and the rhythm stopped.

79

Now I knew we were dealing with something that happened 12 years ago, the latter part of that year, while he was working, involving a male figure and that it created enough fear that it still resided in the tissues of Aaron's lower back muscles.

At this point I induce as much relaxation as possible. I asked Aaron to take two deep breaths, holding them for two counts each and slowly letting the breath out. When this was complete I asked him to journey back into his mind to 1993 (12 years previous to the appointment).

"Do you remember where you were on assignment at that time?" His body began to tense.

"Why?" His eyes flew opened and he looked directly at me with an almost defiant stare.

I closed my eyes and focused on what his body was telling my hands. (I close my eyes because my sensitivity to touch increases when I take away one of the other senses. So I spend much of my time working with my eyes closed. Also I have found that the client is more responsive if I'm not looking at him/her.)

"Because this was apparently a fairly significant time for you or your body wouldn't be bringing it up," I responded.

"But how do you know about that. You don't have clearance for that."

"No, I don't Aaron. And I don't need details that you can't divulge, but I do need you to go back in your mind to that time and answer a few questions so we can release this trauma from your body." I spoke slowly and quietly trying to reassure him it was going to be okay.

"Can you tell me what country you were in?"

"No, not really."

"Because you can't remember or because of confidentiality?"

"Confidentiality."

"Ok, but you do remember where you were and what you were involved in, correct?"

"I remember all my missions. Even the ones I don't want to remember."

"Was this one of those you would rather forget?"

"Yes!"

"When you think back to that mission, who is the first male figure to pop into your mind? Don't over analyze this, just the first one."

"I can't say."

"Just a first name, will do."

"Alexander, Alex."

I needed the name to check against the CSR to make sure we were addressing the correct event and people involved. The CSR indicated yes when he said Alexander.

"Good. And can you tell me what emotion you feel when you think of Alex and that mission?"

I waited but it didn't seem as though Aaron was going to respond. "Aaron?"

"I don't want to talk about it."

"Your conscious mind doesn't want to, but obviously your body needs to address the incident. I see a red pin point of a light, followed by a blast of white light." He said nothing but his breathing was becoming rapid and shallow and his forehead was dotted with beads of sweat.

"Hang in there with me, Aaron. You're doing great." In a soft reassuring voice I said, "Now all I see is black. Can you tell me what these images mean?"

He didn't speak -- just continued to breathe hard and sweat more profusely. In a louder voice I told him to take a deep breath in for five counts, hold for two and release for five. At first there was no response so I repeated the order a little louder and firmer. He immediately took a breath in, held and released. I asked him to do it again, wanting to make sure I had him back here in my room and not in some foreign country with someone named Alex. I also reached up and dabbed his forehead with a Kleenex to wipe away the sweat while maintaining contact with my other hand on the area that held the trauma.

When his breathing had returned to normal and his forehead was clear of sweat I again asked the question, "Can you tell me what the images represent?"

"The red pinpoint was the laser beam on Alex's head, the burst of white was the mussel fire that killed him, and the black was what was left of him. And it all happened on my watch. I was lead. It was my fault." Aaron no longer had the rapid staccato voice of last week or when he arrived for his appointment. He spoke in a flat monotone that reminded me of a flat sheet of dull, grey, ugly metal.

"And how did that make you feel."

"Angry, really angry!"

"Yes, I imagine it would. Did you feel anything else?"

"I shouldn't say what I felt in front of a woman." Pause. "But, I was really, really angry. It shouldn't have happened."

I heard the words Aaron was saying but the tone of his voice did not resonate with the words he was saying and neither did the tissues of his lower back. Remember, that when I asked the questions before starting this release, his body had told me the emotion he was holding was fear. This is often the case. We think we are feeling one thing because it seems more appropriate to us or it is more acceptable in some way, but the true emotion wants acknowledgement. It is the only way we can really process the emotion and release it from our memory, whether it be muscle memory or conscious memory. I needed to bring Aaron's awareness around to what he had felt even deeper than the anger during this event.

"Aaron, when you would go into a mission like that one, where you ever frightened for yourself or your team?"

"Not really for myself, but yes, I felt responsible for getting my team out alive."

"And what about the people you were rescuing? Were you frightened for them?"

"Hmmm, I don't think frightened, just responsible."

"So you only felt responsible, not fear, for both your team and the people you were going after?"

"You can't feel fear. It will destroy you."

I felt like I wasn't getting anywhere with this. Somehow I needed to bring Aaron around to the acknowledgement of fear. But, he had been trained over and over not to feel fear.

"I would feel a great deal of fear each time I went into a situation like that. I would be afraid I wouldn't be able to get my team out safe or fearful that I wouldn't get the person out alive."

"That's because you aren't trained. "

"So you didn't ever feel that way?"

Aaron was quiet. Then he said, "My back really hurts. What are you doing?"

"I'm not doing anything but holding the space. I think your back is trying to tell you something. Just focus on the area that hurts and open your mind to that event."

"I don't think I want to go back there anymore."

"I know, but you need to. Your body needs you to."

A few minutes later, a single tear rolled slowly out of the corner of Aaron's closed eye and down his cheek to his ear. "Yeah, I was afraid. Especially that night, because I knew in my gut the odds were incredibly stacked against us going into that assignment. I wanted to be anywhere but there." The words came out so softly I had to lean in slightly to make sure I heard him. "I knew we probably weren't going to be able to bring Alexander out alive, but I really wanted to, you know. And in that split second that I saw that red bulls eye I was scared to death, because I didn't know where it was coming from and I couldn't get to him no matter how hard I tried. And I tried man, I really tried."

Aaron didn't shed anymore tears. He was trained not to do that. But as he spoke the muscles in his lower back began to soften, ripple and move into their proper position. When they were fully relaxed and the CSR was broad and full, Aaron gave an audible sigh. His whole body began to relax as if the storm had passed and the sun was about to come out again.

After giving him a few minutes for his nervous system to reset and relax, I asked, "What is going on in your life now that parallels that fear? Perhaps on a lesser intensity but, the same type of fear."

"I always feel responsible for everyone and everything. And what if I make a wrong decision? That just isn't acceptable."

"Isn't that being a little hard on yourself? We all make mistakes."

"But when I made a mistake in judgment, someone died."

"Wait a minute, you told me a few minutes ago, that going into that mission you felt the odds were definitely against you being successful. So how did you making a bad decision get Alex killed?"

"I should have sent someone else closer to him then maybe that person could have got Alex out of the way soon enough."

"And maybe it wouldn't have made any difference."

"Maybe but, I will never know so I just have to live with that."

"Is that what you want, is to carry that guilt around with you, when you might not even merit guilt? Cause if that is what you need to do, you can do that."

"I made a poor decision. Someone was killed. I have to live with that."

"Or not."

"You don't understand."

"I understand that you feel that you deserve to pay some undetermined debt to someone because Alex died on an assignment you led. But, let me ask you Aaron, when is the debt paid and who are you paying it to?"

"I don't know. Okay, but what if I make another poor decision? Then what?"

"Hmmm, maybe you'll be human?" I said trying to lighten the moment. "Really, Aaron, is it realistic to think that you can always make the right decision?"

He didn't respond, so I went on. "And on top of that, you are no longer the lead on a hostage rescue team. And most likely no one is going to die just because you make a bad decision whether you are at work or at home. Right? You're making decisions now based on fear. Fear of making a mistake."

"What else do you make them on?"

"At home, based on love. At work, based on good judgment, professional advice, and statistics. Can you give yourself permission to occasionally make a less than optimum decision knowing that you are only human?"

He didn't respond right away. Just lay there with his eyes closed. And then barely audibly he said, "Yes, I think I can."

He began to dose off shortly after that and I finished up the treatment by clearing a couple of other critical points in the cranial system.

I continued to work with Aaron for a total of six appointments a week apart. Most appointments we delved into other events that he was holding onto and examined the emotions he was feeling. Aaron's insomnia improved substantially as did his anxiety. He began to walk at a more normal, relaxed pace and the cadence of his speech slowed down. He was not able to recognize these two changes but, said people at work and his family all commented on them. He found he wasn't as irritable and this was due to the fact that his physical body and his emotional body were coming into alignment as well as the fact that being less critical of himself allowed him to also be more tolerable of those around him.

I continue to see Aaron once every three or four months to clear things out or see what else has come up. But, overall we've gotten him off his medications, his blood pressure is normal, his sleep is good, and his home life is improved.

Post-Traumatic Stress Syndrome whether sustained because of serving in the military or from experiencing a traumatic event in your everyday life has several common factors. A person suffering from PTSD doesn't necessarily suffer from all the symptoms but you will usually see a few of them in the person's life. They are:

- Insomnia
- Hyper-vigilance
- Intrusive thoughts
- Flashbacks
- Panic Attacks
- Long-term fear
- Depression and perhaps suicidal thoughts or attempts

Let's take a look at each one of these symptoms and how CST can help.

Insomnia can result when the joints of the head and neck are jammed together from extreme backward or forward bending of the head (like the action in a whiplash during a rear-end collision or being grabbed from behind in a choke hold). CST is used to release the sutures of the skull releasing this pressure while improving the flow of fluids to and from the brain. This increased fluid to the brain brings nourishment and when it returns from the brain, cleanses and detoxifies the brain.

Hyper-vigilance is a state of heightened awareness. When someone is locked into hyper-vigilance any surprise or unexpected noise causes them to respond excessively and they cannot control their response. (This also contributes to the insomnia problem.) The reticular activating system of the brain and spinal cord is responsible for the secretion of adrenalin and other stress hormones. CST can help reduce this systems action by "dialing down" to normal both the person's hyper-vigilance and also the hyper-responsiveness by bringing homeostasis to the reticular activating system.

Intrusive thoughts continually interrupt a PTSD sufferer's ability to concentrate, sometimes to the point of mental disability. CST is used to balance fluid flow and release restrictions on both the left and right sides of the cranium. Because of this, nutritional supplies can more efficiently and completely reach the brain cells. However, the other important factor is the release of the fluids which carry toxic waste products away from the brain, cleansing it. This allows the parts of the brain that helps control conscious thoughts to be revitalized and function more effective.

Flashbacks are the mental re-visiting of the initial horrific event(s) that are causing the PTSD. Each time the victim has a flashback the event is just as terrifying to the person as the first time. Unlike normal memories, the event does not mellow with each re-visit whether it is through discussion or dreams. (Note when Aaron started recalling the memory he had an intense physical reaction of rapid breathing and profuse sweating.) Often, the person cannot put into words what happened. (Notice Aaron's inability to tell me what had happened until I told him what I saw.) We would expect these types of reactions close to the time of the event(s). However, 12 years later it is not an appropriate reaction, especially being in a safe environment.

Studies have shown that, in PTSD sufferers, the left side of the brain is less functional than the right side. It has also been noted that the part of the brain, (the hippocampus) which plays an important factor in memory control, is smaller on the left side that on the right side. CST helps to equalize the mobility and fluid flow to both sides of the brain. During a session there is significant energy passed from right to left. CST can also focus on the left side which is the predominant speech area of the brain. Emotional release work helps to identify the time and event and release the memory from the tissues so when the brain processes the event the two will come into alignment. Eventually, the power of the event(s) fades and the need for the flashback ceases.

Panic attacks often mark the beginning of PTSD, but they tend to fade or discontinue altogether as the hyper-vigilance, intrusive thoughts and flashbacks are treated.

Long-term fear results in PTSD sufferers who were faced with a short-lived, scary episode in their life. This long term fear eventually becomes anxiety which contributes to the insomnia and the hyper-vigilance. Emotional release work can help the victim identify and release the need for this companion in their life and become more reasonable in the expectation and observance of normal everyday activities. (Like with Aaron who was fearful of making any mistake currently in his life, which was creating anxiety within himself.)

Depression and suicidal thoughts are common among PTSD victims. Often in high achievers these two symptoms are well disguised. CST treatments focus on specifically releasing abnormal compression at three important junctions of the body. The first is where the sphenoid bone (the bone that houses the eyes) and the base of the occipital bone (the large bone at the base of the skull) meet, secondly, where the joints of the first cervical (neck) vertebra and the occipital bone meet, and last, where the lumbar (low back) vertebra and the sacrum (tailbone) come together. These three areas are crucial for keeping the fluids of the body moving benefitting the function of the brain and all the nerves. I know I've said this before, but it is worth repeating, the central nervous system that is being worked with during a CST session governs the entire body, alleviating multiple issues.

In a small study done involving 22 Vietnam veterans, it was found that by doing two weeks of intensive work (3 sessions per week), all of them tested significantly lower on their depression and stress tests. All were experiencing improved sleep habits and all were seeing the benefit of improved concentration. Even the psychologist who was brought in to do the pre and post testing was shocked and had trouble believing the results.

It may be difficult for you to imagine that something so simple to do and to experience could have such profound and meaningful effects on a person's life. You are not alone. I often marvel at the responses I see in people, like Aaron. The body is a remarkable machine that has, at its highest intention, the will to survive. We just need to provide the proper environment and road map for it to get there.

My simple wish is that more people knew about the benefits of CST so they and those they love could be helped from the symptoms of this dreaded syndrome.

Chapter 8

Emotional Pain Becomes Physical Disorder

Lindsay

In a previous chapter we explored the case where Aaron felt violated and suffered stress because of something he witnessed rather than something physical or emotionally done directly to his person. Also, Aaron came from a background (military) where he was used to giving or being given orders or assignments. These cases of PTSD or trauma release and the effect of the trauma are handled slightly different than when dealing with someone who has experienced personally the violation to themselves. Often these people feel the event(s) are beyond their control. They feel as though they have no say in what happened. The trick is to have the client revisit the experience, identify the emotion(s), and *give permission* (by so doing take back control) to release the emotion. This then empowers the victim to overcome and let go of the event(s), as was the case with Lindsay.

You will remember Lindsay that I introduced to you back in chapter 1. If you remember; Lindsay came into my office, a slight young woman in her early 30s. She was definitely underweight by perhaps 10-15 pounds. She seemed like a one dimensional picture, rather than a living breathing person.

First let's review her medical history. She had been diagnosed with fibromyalgia, irritable bowel syndrome, and extensive food and environmental allergies. She had also been diagnosed with depression, but her doctor felt the depression was a response to the fibromyalgia and IBS. Her irritable bowel syndrome coupled with the resulting depression was believed to be the cause of her continual weight loss. She had originally been prescribed Paxil for her depression and fibromyalgia symptoms and Alosetron for the IBS. However, due to the side effects and safety concerns with Alosetron, even though it seemed to help, the doctor took her off it after just a few months.

Now before I go further I want to take a moment to talk about disorders and their titles such as fibromyalgia or chronic fatigue syndrome, or even chronic pain disorder. Many people both in and out of the medical field and the alternative field would argue whether these disorders even really exist. Many people and doctors "poo poo" these disorders or syndromes as made up and that the symptoms those labeled with them are experiencing are really more in their head. My personal belief is that they are constellations of physical symptoms that are very real. However, I believe that the label is a catch all tag for "pain management". The way I treat these clients is to manage their pain and treating the source, not the pain. Also, too often I find the person labeled with the disorder begins to associate themselves with the tag and then they become the disorder. We will go into this and how to break that chain as I share the next couple of case studies.

Back to Lindsay; she was currently off all medications and under the comprehensive care of a naturopathic doctor who had made improvements with her irritable bowel syndrome and allergies but she was still having fairly high levels of pain throughout her body. She was also not gaining weight which was obvious in her bony appearance. She was still having difficulty getting going in the morning and felt "rather bland" as she put it.

I observed her as I welcomed her with a smile and a hand shake. I noticed that as I introduced myself, the smile was returned, the polite words and expressions followed, but the words were hollow, without any emotion. She gave the impression of a doll whose string had been pulled and the replies came out automatically. It seemed rather haunting to encounter this shell of a person who had a name and a history but so little substance. She had been referred to me by her naturopathic doctor to see what I could do about her constant random body pain.

After my observations and a brief explanation of my work we began with the physical part of the session.

As I cradled Lindsay's head in my hands and started the process of observing and listening as I do all appointments, I observed that she had no CSR in her head. I shifted my hands to her shoulders; there was a small trace of rhythm but nothing remarkable. So I shifted my hands to her abdomen and lower back area. Here again there was a noticeable trace but only enough to know when to start moving with the natural rhythm. I began to follow the rhythm and gently nudge it in the direction of ease and it did respond slightly. During the first two appointments with Lindsay the entire time was spent trying to get a healthy CSR going.

On her third appointment with me, she reported no noticeable changes in her body. I asked specifically about pain, quality of sleep, and energy. She shrugged and trying to smile said, "Maybe." This was not the response I was looking for. By this time I had hoped that she would start feeling some pain relief and more energy. As I lay my hands on her again the rhythm was barely perceptible. Knowing I needed to dig deeper and find an underlying issue I asked the body to identify my indicators of yes and no. Once I had the definite stopping of rhythm for yes and speeding up of the rhythm for no I asked if this lack of rhythm and being able to maintain it was being driven by emotions. Her body indicated a profound yes. I then asked the body where it was holding the emotion that was interfering. As I started listing the areas of the body the rhythm stopped on lumbar/abdominal. This made sense when you think about how severe her IBS had been and how she wasn't gaining weight. She probably wasn't digesting or absorbing the foods she was finally able to eat.

I moved my hands to this area and while observing the CSR I asked the body, "When did you first experience the emotion being held here?" Answer: 6 years ago, early part of the year.

"Was there another person involved?" Answer: yes.

"Was it male?" Answer: yes.

"Is it a family member?" Answer: yes.

"What emotion is being held here?" Answer: betrayal.

So I asked Lindsay to take a nice deep breath in and very slowly let it out. When this was complete I asked her to go back in her mind to the year indicated, early in that year and tell me where she was living at the time. She told me the city she had lived in.

"Were you living in an apartment or a house?"

She responded, "A house."

"When you would go into that house was it usually through the front door, a garage or what?"

"Through the garage."

"Ok Lindsay, I'd like for you to see yourself pulling up to the house and opening the garage door. Now get out of the car and go into the house. As you begin to wander through the house, what room are you drawn to stop in?"

It took her a few minutes to go through this and tentatively she asked, "The family room?"

Because she wasn't sure I checked the CSR when she said this to make sure she was on the correct track of remembering what her body needed acknowledged. It indicated, "yes".

"Okay, good. And describe the family room to me. What colors were the walls and carpet, what furnishing, etc."

She proceeded to describe the room to me, telling me about a TV, couch, recliner and a desk with the computer and a chair in front of the desk.

"Ok and is there anywhere you are drawn to sit down or do you prefer to remain standing?"

"Well I would oftentimes check my emails when I got home, because we had recently moved there and I was still missing my family and friends. So I guess I would sit at the computer."

"Ok. As you sit down, a male figure walks into the room. Who is it? The first one that pops into your head."

She didn't answer me. Instead I felt the rigid tissues of her abdomen become even more unyielding. I waited. Then she began to cry. At first it was just a few silent tears creeping out the corners of her eyes, but eventually even though she tried to stop them the tears came rushing out freely. I handed her some tissues and asked again, "Who is it, Lindsay? The first name that came into your mind."

"My husband," she whispered.

"Do you know why you're crying?" (I know this seems like an odd question but often the emotions come to the surface, but, because they have been buried for some time, the client doesn't remember a specific event or reason. They just feel this emotion when they think of that person or event.)

She simply nodded but didn't respond.

"Can we talk about it?" I asked.

"Do I have to? It is kind of humiliating."

"Is that the emotion that you would associate with this person at that moment? You felt humiliated?"

"Ummm, ahhhh," she was struggling. I wasn't sure if she was having a difficult time identifying the emotion or just didn't want to talk.

"Lindsay, this was a rather important turning point in your health. I hope you know I'm here to help you, not judge you or your family. It will help if you can talk to me about it."

"I'm embarrassed," she mumbled.

"Well, I believe everyone is self-conscious at some time or another, and sometimes profoundly embarrassed." I was thinking that she must have done something or said something that she didn't want to tell me.

She was quiet. I waited and then eventually prompted her, "Lindsay".

Then she started talking, the words tumbling out after each other as if she said it quickly enough it would all be forgotten. "He came running into the family room. I mean running down the stairs and into the room. He yelled, Stop! I remember I was so startled I whirled around on the chair so fast I almost fell off. I was so bewildered at the whole thing I didn't even know what I was supposed to stop doing. Then he must have realized how strange he was acting and kind of laughed. But it sounded really odd, almost scary. But it couldn't have been scary because this was my husband. Right?" Without a pause the words ran on, "I remember I was looking at him thinking he was acting really bizarre. This wasn't the first time he had seemed mysterious, but it was by far the oddest he had behaved." She stopped as if frozen in her memory. I prompted her to go on as I observed that her abdomen was beginning to soften up a little so that it felt more like putty than a hard rock.

In a faraway voice that told me she had traveled back in time she went on. "Then he just stood there staring at me. So I turned back around to put my hand on the mouse to wake the monitor up from sleep mode. At that time he moved really quickly and grabbed my hand and yanked my arm around while telling me he wanted to show me something. He had my arm gripped so hard he was hurting me. I told him to let go because he was hurting me and he got all apologetic. It was just really peculiar."

"I asked what he wanted to show me but he just kind of mumbled something so I turned back to the computer and asked if it could wait because I was expecting an email from my sister. But again as I started to reach for the mouse he grabbed my arm and pulled me off the chair. He had never been physical with me before so his behavior shocked me. I think I was afraid of him at that moment. He's so strong from all the personal training he does on base." (Her husband was a Marine on active duty at the time.)

"He hugged me to him and basically ushered me out of the room. But then he just stopped and we stood there. It was as if he was trying to figure out what to do next. I was pretty shaken so I didn't do or say anything, just waited. About that time the telephone rang but we both just continued standing there. Then he gave me a little shove towards the kitchen and told me to go answer it. But I didn't want to talk to anyone so I told him to let the answering machine pick up. I could tell he was getting really frustrated but then we heard his dad's voice on the answering machine, telling him that he knew he was there and to pick up the telephone. So he went to answer it but told me to wait right there. As soon as he was past the doorway I went back to the computer to see what the problem was. I figured he didn't want me seeing whatever it was that was on there."

After a few quiet tears Lindsay whispered, "And he was right not to want me to see."

The tissue in Lindsay's abdomen had been softening and feeling almost normal. However, when she reached this part of the story it immediately seized up again.

It wasn't easy for Lindsay to tell me the whole story. She came from a religious background and was active in her local church. In fact church members had been her support when she left home and went to college and the two times they had been reassigned to new areas. I bring this up because it was significant in how she chose to identify her feelings as being embarrassed at her husband's adultery rather than angry or betrayed. She was afraid that if people in her congregation at church knew they would think less of her as a wife or of her husband.

From here she went on to find that her husband was addicted to pornography and had numerous one night encounters, especially when overseas. He, like many addicts found ways of blaming others and making their addiction someone else's fault, namely her fault. Choosing to be embarrassed allowed Lindsay to not have to take control of the situation or act, but to become further victimized by believing that she was some way at fault. Being a victim freed her from responsibility but it also left her powerless, and cowering for fear others might find out what a pitiful wife and woman she had turned out to be. This was so difficult and painful for her that eventually she chose to become emotionless. Just a shell of a person. She was so powerless and embarrassed that she was killing herself a little at a time by being sick and not able to digest or absorb nutrition. Of course she was doing this unconsciously through a darkened veil of misery and misdirection.

It was critical for Lindsay to be able to identify her true emotions and feelings about herself and her husband in order to bring her physical body (the pain and inability to digest food) and her emotional self (her depression and lack of will to live) into alignment, giving both the acknowledgement they needed in order to heal.

We worked back through the event and I helped Lindsay come to the realization that at the core of all of this the emotion she had buried, but was really feeling was betrayal. Once she was able to identify the true emotion she had felt she agreed she was ready to release the betrayal (she took control) and begin to live again, even though she wasn't sure how to do that. Anne-Schaef Wilson brought this process of recognizing our true emotions and their consequential behaviors to focus when she said, "You need to claim the events of your life to make yourself yours."

We had now followed the long and perverse path back to Lindsay's pain and illness and now the challenge would be finding the bridge that would cross the murky waters of her story to the healing fields of peace and love within herself. This is where I relied upon her own inner wisdom, that I believed knew exactly what she needed to heal far more than I did.

Luckily, Lindsay had been a creative writing major in college and loved to write. Since the birth of her son a little over a year from the onset of her marriage, she had quit working and slowly over time, quit writing. With the discovery of her husband's affairs and his cruel emotional manipulation she had lost all confidence in her ability to do much of anything, including writing. So each week Lindsay would leave my office with encouragement for her to write daily, if only for 10 minutes a day. There is a specific technique I use to help clients access the information hidden within them that will help them to heal. We will discuss this technique later in chapter 12.

Lindsay and I worked for 6 months, first weekly and then as she became stronger both physically and emotionally she developed her own set of tools for dealing with life and we extended the time between visits. As she became stronger emotionally, discovering her love of life and self she began to forgive. The forgiveness process involved far more than her husband. That situation, as is so often the case, is a current day manifestation of issues of a story she had begun to write years previously in her life.

She eventually filed for divorce after attempting various forms of couple therapy. This took a great deal of courage for Lindsay, which she would not have been able to do if she had not reclaimed herself. Ultimately she, like many people recovering from abuse, realized her husband was a sniper. Snipers are deadly. Jody Hayes reminds us, "Snipers are people who undermine your efforts to break unhealthy relationship patterns." He, like all snipers, found her recovery threatening and did whatever he could to sabotage it.

As her emotional well-being improved so did Lindsay's physical symptoms. As long as she avoided the foods she was highly allergic to her IBS was not a problem, even without medication. She began enjoying eating and gained 13 pounds. Due to her ability to absorb her food and nutrients her complexion colored up nicely and her eyes began to shine. There was depth and beauty to this woman who had once been nothing more than an array of skin and bones.

In 2009 while writing an article addressing auto-immune diseases, Dr. Joseph Mercola stated, "The second factor, which is almost universally present in most all auto-immune diseases, (such as the symptoms of Fibromyalgia Lindsay was experiencing) is some kind of predisposing traumatic emotional insult. And unless that specific insult is addressed in some type of effective treatment modality, then the underlying emotional trigger will not be removed, allowing the destructive process to proceed. Therefore, it's very important to have an effective tool to address these underlying emotional traumas."

I agree strongly with Dr. Mercola because it has been my experience that without the emotional insult to the body being resolved, the physical symptoms will continue to scream for attention. It is the primary means by which the physical body gets our attention that something is wrong.

A paper by Joaquín Andrade, M.D., and David Feinstein, Ph.D., summarizes clinical observations involving energy-oriented psychotherapy treatments with 29,000 patients from 11 allied treatment centers in South America during a 14-year period. The paper is entitled "Energy Psychology: Theory, Indications, and Evidence." In addition to the large sample of clinical trials, a number of randomized, double-blind studies were conducted. One of these compared approximately 2,500 anxiety disorder patients who were receiving energy therapy treatments with 2,500 receiving the established treatment for anxiety disorders - medication combined with Cognitive Behavioral Therapy (CBT). The energy psychology treatments were superior to the medication/CBT protocol in the proportion of patients showing some improvement (90% vs. 63%) and the proportion of patients showing complete remission of symptoms (76% vs. 51%). In a related pilot study by the same team, the length of treatment was significantly shorter with energy therapy than with CBT (mean = 3 sessions vs. mean = 15 sessions).

The authors of the article emphasize that these were pilot studies and any conclusions must be considered preliminary and tentative. Nonetheless, the findings are impressive, and they constitute the most persuasive practical support for the efficacy of energy-based psychotherapy to date.

I'm happy to report that I saw Lindsay about a year and a half ago from this writing. She and her son have relocated and started fresh. She is thriving as a freelance writer doing magazine articles. She has been in a mutually rewarding relationship for a year and according to her it has great potential for the future. With a broad, sincere smile that spread clear to her eyes she told me, "I'm finally able to open my heart wide open and let God bless me in whatever way He sees fit. I love being able to sit back and watch the world unfold." Then she handed me a journal with the following inscription,

Dear Annette,

A wise woman once encouraged me to write for 5 – 10 minutes every day and to ask myself, "What I need to do to……. (finish the sentence)."

This small gift of mine is a little reminder for the story you want to tell but can't seem to write.

With love and appreciation, Lindsay

And so now I write back to Lindsay, "Thank you for encouraging me to write this book. Thank you for taking the responsibility of healing emotionally and physically. And thank you for letting me be a part of that process."

Chapter 9

The Complex World of Addiction

Lisa

In the previous case studies I have focused on the primary issue the client presented with in my office. However, with this next case study I am going to go into great length to detail out the multiple issues that can be found in a single client. Most clients, even those I've shared with you already, had various matters in their lives that needed adjustments; such as life style choices, family issues, and even addictions. Please bear with me as we explore Lisa's multifaceted life. I feel there is much to be learned from the dynamics of this case study.

Lisa was a 40 year old, stunningly beautiful brunette who I happened to meet publicly at a small social gathering one evening. She was the sister-in-law of Adam, my date for the evening. It didn't take me long to realize two things about Lisa. One, she had a wickedly biting tongue that she didn't hesitate to use and, two, that there was little affection whatsoever between her and Adam. She knew exactly what buttons to push on him and did not hesitate to do it -- even though we were in a small but relatively private setting and he was with someone she had never met before. The other observation, an easy one to make, was the amount of alcohol Lisa was consuming and the obvious embarrassment Adam's brother, Wes, and their two children were suffering at her lack of self-restraint.

The evening was rather awkward, and I wondered if I would ever have the experience of seeing Lisa again. Even though I was uncomfortable with her belligerent behavior I have dealt with enough people who are aching to recognize she was hurting with a capital "H". I felt empathy for her, a woman who was so desperately calling out for attention in all the wrong ways.

A few weeks later, Adam's parents hosted a bonfire to burn off the autumn leaves and debris at their family ranch. Adam called me and somewhat sheepishly asked if I thought I could handle another one of his family adventures. "Since they are so much fun," he said sarcastically. "I would completely understand if you say 'no.' I would say no if I thought I could get away with it." Then softness came into his voice as he finished, "But Mom would be disappointed if I wasn't there."

The odd thing was that Adam and his parents had a wonderfully endearing relationship and enjoyed each other's company. I had observed this a couple of times and could hear it in Adam's voice when he spoke of them. He also spoke fondly of his brother, Wes, and their times growing up. So it seemed odd that he had such dread for family gatherings.

The old fashioned bonfire, complete with a ghost story and s'mores was great fun. However, there was Lisa and she could not find a single enjoyable thing about the evening. She complained about the smoke, the logs were too hard to sit on, the food had too much fat, she couldn't even think of eating a s'more because of the calories. Early into the evening she excused herself, complaining of a headache and walked back up to the house. Wes followed her and they had a discussion, which I could not hear but that obviously became heated judging by the tone of their voices. When Wes returned and sat down on the log next to Adam and me, he put his head in his hands and just slouched there with slumped shoulders.

"You have got to do something about her, Wes. You and the kids can't keep going through this," said Adam softly, so he wouldn't be heard by the others.

Wes lifted his head, looked directly at his brother with utter hopelessness and said, "Yeah, like what? We've had her in two different rehab programs. They work just long enough to give the family a little hope for some kind of normal future and so that you don't think you totally wasted those thousands of dollars." He put his head back in his hands and said quietly, "But it never lasts. She always goes back to the alcohol. I don't think there *is* a fix."

"Then you need to get out of this situation. It isn't healthy for you or the kids. Look at you -- you've lost weight and your aging way too fast."

"Well, thanks for all the encouraging words, Brother." He meant these words to be sarcastic, but there was no fire behind them. Only sadness. After a pause he raised his head again, looked first at me and then at Adam and said, "But is that really the answer. She is the mother of my children. "And," his voice dropped off then as if he was far away, "I remember when it was good. It was good in the beginning and I really loved her. I just want that back. Is that too much to ask?"

Often I run into people and their families that are this discouraged. They spend thousands of dollars going from one doctor or therapist to another looking for the cure to what ails them. They are doing the best they can for themselves or their loved ones with the options they know about. Most of the time they don't know how closely the emotions and the physical body are entwined. They especially don't know that the physical body can be used to access the emotions that are keeping them from moving on in their lives and overcoming addictions or chronic issues.

I had sat listening to this exchange not wanting to interfere with what was obviously a very personal discussion between these two brothers. But when I heard the familiar plea for help and total desperation in Wes' voice, I couldn't stay silent any longer. "I don't know what you've tried in the past, but what I do know about addiction is that it is a multi-faceted disease. There is a physical side to it. Her body has obviously been worn down and is now starving for healthy nutrients.

However, because of her strong need to not feel, she chooses alcohol over healthier choices. Then there is the emotional/spiritual side of the disease. She is screaming for help."

Before I could go on Adam broke in angrily. "Wait a minute. Wes has offered her help from early on. And so have my parents. They have been there all along, putting up with her hurtful behavior and never criticizing or judging her or Wes. So don't give me a sob story about poor Lisa 'screaming for help.' I just don't buy it."

The sudden amount of venom in Adam's tone surprised me. This was a part of him I had not witnessed before. I looked to see what Wes' reaction was to this outburst. What I saw on Wes's face and in his whole body language was not appreciation for his brother's loyalty and support but shame and guilt for what he was putting both his family and his extended family through. As in so many cases, the effects of the addiction spread out like a ripple in a pond of water. What starts as a pebble (the actions of the addicted person) eventually spreads out and changes the lives, emotions and actions of anyone in its wake.

I placed a reassuring hand on Adam's knee to communicate to him I understood how he felt, but at the same time needed to finish what I was saying. "I don't doubt that all of you have tried to be supportive and loving. I don't doubt that you, Wes, have spent untold amounts of money on trying to help her. But you both have to admit she is still crying out for something."

"Yeah, *attention*," said Adam flatly. I could tell he wasn't happy with me and what he perceived as a lack of allegiance. He had shifted his body away from me and now he shrugged my hand off his knee, stood, and started to pace. "I'm just concerned for Wes and the kids. She's burned bridges with me too many times." This explained a lot to me about why he dreaded family gatherings. None of us feel comfortable going into situations where there are unresolved judgments and resentments. But again, this conversation was about Lisa, not Adam, so I continued.

"Has she ever had body work to address the emotional issues that she's hanging on to?" I asked Wes.

"She's had so many hours of counseling I couldn't even begin to tell you how many or what technique they used. She has gone to a number of people. She gets massages every couple of weeks, too. The counselors told her that might help. Helps drain my pocket book, I know that."

"There is a multi-facetted way of treating this disease that you probably haven't done before if you have relied on the

108

traditional medical model," I told Wes. Adam stopped pacing now and, looking skeptical, he stood in front of me.

"Shall we call in the astrologers, the psychics or maybe the witches? Yep just bring in the kooks. I don't suppose you've tried that before have you, Wes?" asked Adam – again, so sarcastically I was taken aback.

We had not discussed in any detail what I specifically did with my clients because it is so difficult to explain to people who have never experienced alternative medicine or have tried one technique and not seen any results. So Adam didn't realize how personal his words were. But again, he was the one in the ripple, and I needed to address the needs of pebble that caused the ripple.

"What is with you, Adam? You don't have to attack Annette just because she's trying to help," commented Wes.

This was a typical type of response people who are frustrated and unaware of the benefits and the research of alternative medicine. I've dealt with this enough in my profession to know it is best to address it right up front so the person can see that I am comfortable with and understand their attitudes.

"Actually, Adam, it isn't witchery or astrology or anything mystical. There are techniques that use the physical pulses of the body to unblock buried memory. It is actually very similar to the techniques used with lie detector tests. There is also a highly sophisticated computer program that will show the therapist and the doctor exactly what is going on in Lisa's body on an energetic level before it will even show up on a blood test. There has been research and studies completed to show that this form of approach works better than the traditional western medicine model when dealing with chronic issues."

I was grateful for Wes' previous support which encouraged me to continue.

Turning so I was now looking straight at Wes I went on, "It could be that Lisa doesn't even remember the events that are bringing her so much pain. Or she remembers them but has processed them with the understanding of a child. If that is when the events happened to her and now she builds her life on that story rather than a healthy one. I know it's difficult to grasp what I'm saying, but there are forms of bodywork specifically designed to read what the body is saying and holding on to that will allow the therapist to bypass the conscious mind which is confused right now."

"Are you talking about hypnosis?" asked Wes.

"No. It isn't hypnosis. Even though hypnosis can be very valuable, I feel like someone with Lisa's history of treatments would get further faster with the body telling us what needs resolved. Plus I think she might be more receptive to this form of treatment than hypnosis."

"And how much is this going to cost? Shall he put his house up for sale now?" complained Adam.

What Treatment Involves

It could have been easy to become offended by Adam's attitude. If any of you have been in a situation where you or someone close to you has been through multiple treatments and ended up back at the beginning, then you understand the resentment and frustration that Adam was feeling. I had witnessed many clients go through trying circumstances like these, and I did understand.

What often times is not understood by the family members is that their feelings and attitudes often keep the ill or injured person stuck. Even if the ill person, Lisa in this situation, were to get help and start to make improvements, the unconstructive emotions of doubt, fear, and irritation of the others in the family would eventually pull her back into her role in the group. Therefore, without even realizing it they have become part of the problem.

"Considering the enormous cost of personal rehab in a private hospital which I'm assuming costs thousands a day," I paused looking questioningly at Wes for confirmation, which he gave with a roll of his eyes and a resigned nod of the head, "it ranges from $100 per session with the therapist up to $500 with the doctor and the vitamin IVs, supplements and such."

I knew I was treading on thin ice with this situation. Lisa needed help. I felt I could help her. But it is always a balancing act in regards to boundaries when you know someone socially and then they become your client. A therapist needs to keep a healthy boundary between herself and every client so that the client does not become confused about their own ability to heal themselves. They need to be empowered, not become dependent or feel manipulated by the therapist. But, also the therapist needs to not get involved in the client's personal life so that she can remain unattached emotionally to the healing process. Otherwise she risks possibly trying to dictate or manipulate the process. Staying neutral and staying out of the way of the healing process is critical in this work. Mind you, this doesn't mean that I as the therapist I don't care. I care deeply about each of my clients and their healing process, but it is of utmost importance that I not be invested in any particular outcome or I risk taking away their choices in the process.

At this time, I was asking myself, could I truly offer this therapy and maintain the necessary boundaries with Lisa and her family. Hoping that I could, I went on to explain.

111

What the Therapy Would Necessitate

"Coinciding with this therapy she would need to have her physical needs addressed with her receiving intravenous vitamin and amino acid therapy. She would need to be taking some homeopathic remedies and have her nutritional intake evaluated for allergies and absorption. She would also need to be detoxing her body. This would best be done using a far-infra-red sauna, so her liver and kidneys aren't being stressed any more than they are currently. She would have to be evaluated by a physician who would determine whether she can do this outpatient or whether she needs to be in-house for a while. As you've probably figured out, Wes, addiction takes hold of the whole person, inside and out. But if the person is willing to do all the aspects of the treatment totally, I've seen it make an amazing difference in their life."

I did not mention this to Wes at the time -- it would come up soon enough -- but it is important to mention here that addiction is challenging to treat for another reason. Not only is it multi-faceted for the client, but it is also necessary to address the healing process of the family. By the time someone realizes and admits they have an addiction, painful family histories and behaviors have developed. Anyone who closely deals with the addicted on a regular basis has learned compensatory behaviors, just as the body learns to compensate for another part of the body that isn't functioning properly. If these behaviors are not brought to a conscious level of all participants and corrected the addicted will eventually, most likely start playing her/his role again in the family story. This is just like a physical injury that heals, only to keep reappearing because the root issue and compensation patterns aren't fully corrected. They eventually pull the physical body back into poor bio-mechanics and the injury or pain reappears.

Where Was Lisa?

The fire was burning down and most everyone had returned to the house. It was getting late and Adam and I needed to get on the road. We agreed I would send Wes some information and he could think it over. Only later would Adam and I learn that when Wes went upstairs to get Lisa, who'd told him she was going to lie down because of a headache, he found her passed out from alcohol consumption, which she had taken from his parents' bar.

Two days later Adam called to tell me what had happened and explain that Lisa had asked Wes to take her back to the private hospital for rehab. She admitted that she wanted to die. She couldn't go on with the guilt and self-loathing. They were both concerned about her mental well-being and whether she might try to commit suicide. Neither could live with that so they felt committing her to an in-house rehab situation was the best. The children had not had much to say; they were also getting used to this dysfunction.

Ten days later Lisa was released to the care of a physician I work with -- a Family Practitioner who is also a Holistic Healthcare Doctor -- for examination and coordination of her IV vitamin and amino acid therapy, her nutritional intake, allergies, absorption, hormone evaluation, herbs and homeopathic remedies. Once that workup was completed and she had her first infusion, Lisa and I began to work together.

At first she was hesitant... for three reasons. First, she was concerned about my relationship with her brother-in-law and how that would come into play with her privacy and also my judgments of her behavior to date. I told her it would not come into play and that her privacy was sacred to me. I also assured her that who she was last year, and two weeks before, as well as who she was now and who she would become, are all different people, so there was no need for me to judge any of them.

Her second concern was that this was totally new to her and she was nervous not only about the process, but also about what we might discover. People are so invested in who they believe they are and what has made them that way that the mere thought that it could change is frightening. I reassured her of the process and told her I had experienced letting go of my preconceived self too. Once I started realizing I had the power to change things it was a freeing, not frightening experience.

Third, Lisa was desperately afraid of not being successful and letting her family, especially Wes, down again. "I truly think he will leave me if I am not successful this time. And I don't know what I would do without him and the children." There was so much desperation in her voice I wanted to reassure her that would never happen. But, of course, I don't know what will happen in anyone's future. I could only encourage her to use that fear to help her be 100% compliant with her treatments and therapy.

Lisa's First Sign of Hope

The first two hands-on sessions with Lisa were unremarkable. She had a few major restrictions in her system and only two noteworthy restrictions, one in her abdomen and one at the base of her skull. Both released nicely on the first appointment. However, when she returned for her second appointment the restriction in her abdominal region had returned to the same degree. It released easily and the tissues were soft and subtle. She reported sleeping very well after her first appointment, so we requested that her sleep medication be reduced in dosage. That request was granted and she continued sleeping well until her second appointment. Again we requested a reduction in the dosage and this time it was recommended since she was doing so well and the dosage was already low that she discontinues this medication.

By the time Lisa arrived for her third session with me, she had been out of the hospital 28 days. She'd had four intravenous vitamin and amino acid infusions, had been off sleep medication for five days, and felt she was ready to reduce her anti-depressant because she was feeling good. When I pressed her a little for what "good" meant she replied, "I'm coping really well. I don't feel nearly as anxious as in the past, and I don't feel like I want a drink. In fact, I actually am starting to think this might work."

This was the first time I'd heard hope in Lisa's voice since I met her and it was as refreshing as a light summer rain that clears dust from the air, leaving in its wake the desire to take a deep breath.

With that exciting statement and its confirming body language, we began our third session. As I cradled Lisa's head in my hands and settled in to understand what it was her body needed from us today, my attention was immediately drawn, once again, to the restrictions locking up her pelvis and originating in the abdominal region. I asked myself, and Lisa's inner guidance, what this was all about. Why did it keep returning? Then I listened. Nothing in particular came to me and when I asked if the reoccurrence was driven primarily by emotions I couldn't seem to get a definite *yes* or *no*. When asked if it was primarily physical the response was the same. Nothing definite. When this happens, there is another aspect of my work that comes up for me.

Patience, Work…and Added Help

What I have learned through my years of experience is that some traumas in people's lives are so terrible that the person completely locks them away so that their conscious mind will not have to remember or deal with the memories. If they are buried deep enough and long enough it takes patience and prodding from the therapist to get the subconscious to reveal the memories.

This is when I turn to a higher power than myself to do the work. I realize not everyone believes in God. You don't have to in order for the work to progress. I try to be diligent in honoring the client's personal belief system, and if we need to discuss the spiritual path I try to phrase the guidance within their belief system. As for me I am a Christian and have a close and personal relationship with God. I believe that being able to do this work at the level I do and help people heal is a gift God has given me. So when I am stumped or stalled out, I turn to the source of my gift and ask for help.

It is then – **when I open to direction from beyond myself**---that I receive information about the person on my table. Again, I am not psychic and cannot predict the future for anyone. I can only say that at times I seem to receive information. This data usually comes through simply knowing what to do or say next or I will see images. (Remember Aaron, the retired military man with PTSD? When I was working on him, I saw the red pinpoint of light, the flash of white light and then a dense blackness. I can't tell you how I saw those images, only that I needed to see them so I could help Aaron discuss them and help him heal, so they became vivid images in my mind's eye.) This is why doing this work produces such remarkable results for people, like Aaron or Lisa, who are going through PTSD and whose conscious minds won't or can't allow them to talk about their trauma. I can see it and I can say it for them. The other interesting aspect about this part of my work, which I call the spiritual aspect, is that I only get this knowledge when I have my hands on a person's body. The information comes through me touching them.

Returning to Lisa's session...

I waited patiently with my entire focus on the area of Lisa's abdomen that was restricted. Eventually the sensation I became aware of was one of thick dark fog. The type of fog you don't want to drive through for fear of running into something or someone that you can't see soon enough to stop before hitting them.

My first impression was to not go there, but as I stayed with it for another moment the fog began to thin slightly and I could barely make out the silhouette of a man. I got a sinking feeling in the pit of my stomach, like when you are on a roller coaster, climbing the hill part of the track. You have that half-excitement/half-dread feeling because you know very soon your stomach will be in your throat. Again, I stayed with the feeling and the focus but the only other image that came to me was of a young girl, maybe 10 years old. Because of this image I decided to make inquiries of her body as if I knew there was an emotional premise to the restriction.

"When did you first feel the emotion being held in the abdomen?" What came back was, *Age 8.* Next I asked if it involved another person. There was no clear answer so I asked if it involved the man I saw? The rhythm indicated *yes.* Is this related to home life? Again the rhythm indicated *yes.* What emotion are you holding onto? *Humiliation.* I felt I knew where this inquiry was going to take us, and I dreaded it. However, the body had trusted me enough to give me this much information so I could not let it down by quitting or moving on to something else. At this moment I asked for divine guidance and assistance.

After asking Lisa to take a couple of nice deep breaths I asked her to go back in her mind and picture herself as an 8 year old girl. She was quiet, so I inquired if she could remember a picture of herself at that age or close to it. She said she did. I then began taking her back to that time by having her give me more details. What are you wearing in the picture? Is your hair short or long? Were you tall or short for your age? As she described in detail to me the young girl a picture emerged clearly in my mind. I then asked her if she could remember the house where she lived at that time. She indicated she did. We were lucky; she had only lived in one house from birth through high school. So I asked her to describe the outside of the house for me. "Did you usually enter the house through the front door, back door or garage?"

"Garage," she replied in a relaxed almost dreamy voice. This was good. I could tell from her voice and tranquil body language that she was going back in time.

"Okay, Lisa, I want you to see yourself opening the door from the garage and walking into the house. As you do this what room would you like to go into?"

Almost immediately she responded, "My bedroom. I love my bedroom. It was pink and white with a canopy over my bed that I used to pretend was a carriage. I was the princess and I would ride to the ball in my carriage." As she said this I had my eyes closed and most of my focus on the tissues between my hands, but I knew without even looking that Lisa was smiling at this fond memory. "I remember the day I decided my room was too childish and wanted to make it a teenage room." She was moving away from the important moment, so I intervened. I needed to keep her at age 8 for the time being.

"Let's stay with the room the way it was when you were eight years old. So was your room a safe place for you to be?" I asked, wanting to get her back into the moment.

She started to say something but stopped. Then rather hesitantly she whispered, "Yes." I was closely monitoring the tissues as we spoke and all of a sudden the CSR which had been slow and steady sped up and became erratic. The body was telling me that what Lisa was telling me was not in resonance with the body. This is where the conscious and subconscious were diverting to travel the separate paths they had all these years.

"What made you feel safe in your room?" I prodded.

"I don't know. Maybe, well," as Lisa struggled to find an appropriate answer to keep her false memory alive her voice began to take on a child's tone.

After I felt Lisa's focus was sufficiently present in her room I asked Lisa to tell me the name of the first male figure that came into her mind. Then I waited for Lisa to focus her mind.

In only a minute or two, Lisa started feeling hot. Her hands began to sweat and her breathing tempo crept faster as the breath became shallow. "Tell me what you are sensing," I coaxed quietly.

Tears slowly started slipping down Lisa's face from the corners of her eyes as she slowly shook her head no. "It is okay Lisa, I am here with you," I reassured her.

Lisa's Break Through

"No! No! No!" said Lisa. But her tone was more frightened than emphatic. "Please, no," she wailed. Then suddenly she turned on her side and curled into a fetal position. I continued to hold the area of tension, moving with Lisa. I switched techniques to an acupressure hold maintaining contact with the tension in her abdomen with my top hand and a specific point on her lower back with my bottom hand. I needed to be able to constantly monitor the tissues and what her body was directing me to do.

"Lisa, please tell me what you are sensing. I can help you with this." As I waited for her to respond I sent up a silent prayer. *Help me to know what to do and what to say. Please direct my intuition and my hands that we might be able to bring peace to Lisa.* Then I waited some more.

The Body Reveals Its Secrets...When It Is Ready

Let me interject something here. As I scroll through the directory of the Upledger institute there are hundreds of practitioners who have studied the first level of Craniosacral Therapy. But there are much fewer, perhaps about twenty percent, that go on to take the second and more advanced classes. When I've asked practitioners about this and why they aren't using this valuable tool the response is always similar. "It is too slow and boring. I found myself falling asleep." But the fact is this work – the kind I was doing with Lisa – **cannot be rushed**. Whether it is on the physical level or the emotional level, the body has to process at its own speed. Also, as a therapist I have to be willing to wait to receive information when I'm not sure where to go, rather it is coming from the client's body or from a higher source. I act as the facilitator not the director in this unveiling process. Whereas, as a massage therapist, a doctor or a chiropractor, the practitioner is usually trying to get the body to do what they want, with Craniosacral Therapy, I wait for the body to tell me what it needs and how it will get there, and then I facilitate it through that development.

Fortunately, Lisa's physical being had held onto its secret long enough, and now she was ready to reveal it.

Past Abuse

"He hurt me," Lisa said in a small voice barely audible. "He told me I deserved it because I was so pretty. That I wanted him to do it." Lisa's tears had nearly stilled, and this last part was said between hiccups as she tried to regain her composure. But her high-pitched, small voice indicated that she had mentally and emotionally become that 8 year old child again.

This was the information I had expected would come. In the two previous sessions I had gotten minor emotional responses from Lisa. However, it is my experience that when dealing with depression, addictions and/or long term chronic pain there are usually deep emotional wounds that need to be recognized and healed. The response I had elicited from Lisa's body today of curling into the fetal position, voice changes and steady tears all pointed towards my theory as well. Now the trick was to get Lisa's conscious mind to register the event and process it with a perspective equivalent to Lisa's adult mind.

"Lisa, who hurt you?" I asked gently. I was concentrating intently on Lisa's physical body and what its responses were telling me as well as what Lisa was verbalizing. After a few minutes I asked a second time, "Who hurt you, Lisa?"

"I can't tell you. He will cut my face if I tell you," she whispered.

At 8 years old, Lisa was at a very impressionable age and would have fully believed an adult if they told her that.

"I won't let him hurt you again, Lisa. You aren't eight years old anymore. You can tell me who it was." I used a quiet but firm voice, but Lisa only curled tighter into her position.

"He's coming again. I want him to go away. Please make him go away."

"Lisa, you can make him go away. What can you do to make him go away?" I asked.

"No I can't. He has a knife. He will cut me up if I don't do what he wants." With this she started shaking and crying hard, almost hysterically.

I closely monitored how the area of tension in the abdomen was changing. The hard tight knot was finally starting to move. The last thing I wanted to do was discontinue this line of inquiry with Lisa and drive the memory deeper into her subconscious mind to do more damage but I had to be careful not to lose her to the trauma.

"Lisa, you are doing great work. This may be frightening, and it hurts, but it's very positive work. You need to take a deep breath in, hold it for four counts and then slowly let it out. *Okay, big deep breath in.*"

No response.

So louder and with more authority I repeated the request.

In response, Lisa just covered her head with her hands and repeated, "I won't, I won't."

I realized this memory and the emotions it triggered could easily go too far causing her to become hysterical and require medical intervention. On the other hand she was so close and I didn't want to stop her at this point.

So – first, I prayed. Then I concentrated on the message the physical body was giving me. The tissues seemed ready to continue unwinding.

"Lisa, this is Annette," I pressed on gently. "Do you hear me? Do you hear me, Lisa?" My face was right next to Lisa's right ear.

Slowly Lisa began to relax a small amount. Then slowly she nodded her head.

"Good, Lisa, now I need to know if you trust me. This is *Annette*. Do you trust me Lisa?"

Again , she nodded. I took a deep breath. I was perspiring from the heat being given off by Lisa's body and the physical exertion I was expending – and from the tension of the moment. "Now then, Lisa, you trust me so you can tell me who hurt you so I can help you. Who hurt you?" I persisted.

This was critical information especially for Lisa to acknowledge.

"Uncle Rick," she whispered in the small high pitched eight year old voice. "He made me, he made me," she couldn't continue but burst into tears. The tension had been released and the abdominal tissue was soft and subtle. I released the hold on the area and stroked Lisa's back trying to comfort and reassure her.

"I know, I know. It's okay. You don't have to say it," I said softly against Lisa's head. I knew she knew what had happened in her carriage sanctuary those many years ago. I had seen it in my mind's eye and her body's release of the tension convinced me she had processed the events. I gently helped Lisa sit up and cradled her against me until her sobbing subsided. Once Lisa's breathing was under control I asked, "You've never told anyone that before have you Lisa?"

"No! In fact I don't think I even remembered it, until now," she replied slowly.

"Do you feel like continuing or have you had enough for today?" I asked, but Lisa only shrugged her shoulders. So I continued, "I'd like to finish this if you feel up to it."

Without saying anything Lisa lay back down on the table. I walked her through the scenario again this time helping Lisa change the outcome. In this ending she was able to kick him hard and run screaming for help. We visualized this new ending in detail until her body softened and seemed to accept it as a reality.

www.Helpguide.org/mental/emotional_psycological_trauma defines this therapy as "**Somatic experiencing** which takes advantage of the body's unique ability to heal itself. The focus of therapy is on bodily sensations, rather than thoughts and memories about the event. By concentrating on what's happening in your body, you gradually get in touch with trauma-related energy and tension. From there, your natural survival instincts take over, safely releasing this pent-up energy through shaking, crying, and other forms of physical release."

Therefore, we continued to replay the scenario in Lisa's mind with the different ending until her body no longer responded physically to the memory. We know at this point the memory has healed in the tissues themselves and can now be dealt with by Lisa's adult consciousness.

Life Patterns

After we'd re-envisioned Lisa's life, there was a definite change in her energy. She was less tense and more open.

We went on to discuss how this incident had set the pattern for the rest of Lisa's life. She was humiliated and felt helpless and worthless. She felt she was only of value because of her physical beauty. In this frame of mind she actually detested her beauty because she believed her looks had been the cause of the molestation.

I found another area in Lisa's neck where she was holding tension from ten years ago. As I mentioned this date to Lisa she immediately remembered a vicious argument she had with Wes. She had wanted to go to a party that some friends were hosting. Wes had said he would be home to go with her. But, just before he was supposed to be home he telephoned and said that he wasn't going to be able to go. She was angry with him and they fought over the telephone. She decided she was going to go anyway. When she arrived at the party another man was there alone. He made a pass at Lisa trapping her in a corner of the hall. She panicked. She left the party immediately, went home and got drunk. When Wes arrived home he found her passed out and they fought again the next morning.

"This has been the story of my life over and over and over again," wailed Lisa. The tears had started again. I let her cry until the neck area started to relax. Then I asked Lisa to look at that scenario in light of what we now knew about her past.

"Why did the man come on to you?"

"He said because I was so beautiful. I hate being pretty!" she stated emphatically.

"No you don't." I laughed as she said this. "You just hate the louts that think they can touch you because of your beauty."

"That's for sure," Lisa said and sounded much better. I knew a little humor is always good for the soul, especially in highly emotional sessions like this one today.

"Who did this man represent from your past?" I asked.

"Uncle Rick," Lisa said in a quiet unsure voice.

"That is right. Now who did Wes represent?"

After a few minutes Lisa said she wasn't sure.

"Who should have protected you from Uncle Rick?" I asked.

"My dad. Rick was his stinking brother. He should have known, but, no, Dad just kept inviting him over. I hated him!" There was deep seated emotion in her voice.

"Who did you hate, Lisa?"

"*Both* of them," she finally said reverting into that now familiar 8 year old voice.

"Who did Wes represent from your past?" I asked again.

"Daddy," came the little voice.

"And how did you feel about Wes at that time?" I prodded.

"He should have been there. He should have protected me from that creep. But he didn't. He was too busy. So I just showed him. I got stinking drunk because he hates it when I get drunk," said Lisa angrily.

I let Lisa feel this anger until the tissues in her neck were completely relaxed and the CSR was long and expansive; indicating she had acknowledged and processed the emotion, as well as, the connection of people to the roles they'd played. I was also using this time to confirm or deny rather this was the true emotion she was feeling. I then continued, "But how did you really feel inside. Were you mostly angry?"

"Yes, I was furious."

"*Focus* Lisa," I suggested, "*right here* were my hands are on your neck." Then in a quiet still voice I asked again, "What were you really feeling, Lisa?" Her body began to tremble and the tears began to flow again.

"Worthless, humiliated, helpless. What was I supposed to do? The man I loved was too busy for me. This creep had his hands all over me. All I wanted was to be loved."

"By whom?" I asked.

"By *Wes*." She paused and then again in the young girl's voice the real answer, "by Daddy."

"I know what I'm going to tell you isn't as good right now Lisa, but what I want you to know is that God loves you. Wes loves you and I love you. Of all of those loves, God's love is unconditional and constant. You will need to know that for yourself soon in order to overcome this trauma in your life."

Believing in God or a higher source is often difficult for people who have suffered traumas inflicted upon them. In fact they often resent the mention of a God or higher power, feeling that this higher power or God should have protected them. On the other hand, it is my experience with these kinds of horrific traumas that it takes the ability of turning the whole thing over to a higher source that provides complete

127

healing to take place. So we will address this issue in an upcoming section.

Going On From Here.....

I initiated a still point in the cranial system to induce deep relaxation of the body and indicating to the body that we were finished for today. I waited for Lisa's breathing to become slow and deep. I told Lisa we were finished for today and congratulated her on her great work.

"Wow!" was all Lisa said when she sat up. "I am exhausted."

"You deserve to be. Your body did an enormous amount of releasing today which works the metabolic system of the body. It is as if you had run several miles," I reassured.

"That's what it feels like," smiled Lisa weakly. "Thank you. Thank you for being there for me. This is incredible."

As a side note, people need to realize healing is hard physical work on the physiological systems of the body. There needs to be a period of rest and pampering that follows any craniosacral session but particularly one with emotional release work.

Finding The Gift

This life we have chosen to participate in is a rather interesting coalition of people and events. At one point or another most people ask themselves, "Why am I here", "Where did I come from", "What will happen to me after I die"? I believe it is these three weighty questions that help us to delve deeper into life and try to make meaning out of the ciaos we call existence.

It is not the purpose of this book to answer these questions, however, in many of my sessions with clients one, two or all three of these questions will arise at some point in their therapy. This is especially true with clients dealing with emotional trauma, like Lisa. These three questions are tricky enough for the general populace to answer, but for those whose core care givers or loved ones have abused them, the questions can seem impossible to answer.

I'm often asked, "If there is a God, then how could he have allowed this to happen to me?" Or "If there is a God, why does he let bad things happen to good people?" This is a legitimate question. Once you understand a core part of healing it is much easier to understand the answer to these questions.

In every tragedy there is a gift. **I know this is difficult to fathom**. How can there be any gift for Lisa, who was sexually abused as an 8 year old child? How can there be a gift in the trauma of Lisa's father perpetuating the problem by constantly inviting his brother into the home which therefore allowed this horrible situation to continue? With these situations, and others just as horrific it can be very challenging to find the gift. But I promise you, the gift, or often the gifts, are there waiting to be discovered like the long ago lost and buried treasures of the sea. And once they are discovered, and received, they are far more valuable than any chest of gold coins. These gifts become the tools that propel the person to not only recover, but gives them a strength and an understanding that they can rely on whenever the need arises in the future, allowing them to evolve and grow into the person they desire to become.

Again, I'm going to ask you to erase the concrete walls of your previous beliefs and explore with me a different possibility. And that is all it is, a possibility, so you can let your guard down and open your mind to what might be. Suppose we lived in a previous existence, the concept of that existence can be whatever your mind is comfortable with. Imagine that in this previous existence God (in whatever form you are at ease with) had a plan for you. He knew what you would need to learn in this life time here on earth and how you would best learn this personality trait or knowledge. Let's take Lisa for example. God knew this wonderful female lacked certain qualities that she would need to progress. She seemed to lack self-confidence as well as a sense of self. She would need to learn to be strong from the inside no matter what was happening outside of her. She also needed to learn how to be true to herself and her emotions instead of acquiescing to everyone and everything else. But above all she needed to learn in this earth life to trust her instincts and to trust in God.

So knowing this about Lisa, God then needed to create a life or a scenario that would help her to learn these lessons. People were placed in her life that would play roles and create situations where she would have the opportunity, should she choose, to learn these valuable traits.

God already knew the choices that Lisa's uncle had made in the existence he was currently in and how that would determine the types of choices he would make in the earthly existence we are currently in. He therefore placed this man in Lisa's family and allowed him to continue to make choices according to his agency. Through this series of events God was allowing the uncle to make choices for which he would be held accountable, but also giving Lisa an opportunity to learn the important lessons she needed in her existence.

An ancient teaching says, "The world is a teacher to the wise man and an enemy to the fool." I like the way Debbie Ford puts it in her book *The Dark Side Of The Light Chasers*, when she states, "No event is painful in and of itself. It's a matter of perspective. It's important to understand that everything happening in the world is as it should be at every moment."

If you can allow for this scenario in Lisa's life then you can also see where along the way God also placed people in her life that could help her deal with and heal from the trauma while developing the traits she needed. However, Lisa, like most of us, often overlooked these helpful and loving people and situations that were placed in her path and chose pain and destructive behavior until she couldn't take it any longer. It seems to be at these moments of intense discomfort that we finally become humbled by our own misery and/or physical pains that God once again puts someone in our path that will help us start the climb out of our darkness.

As Lisa and I went back over her life she was able to recall a few situations where healing could have begun if she had taken the step but each time chose to turn from the opportunity. Soon after the first event with her uncle her mother noticed bruising on her daughter and questioned her about it. Her mother had always shown her love and kindness, but Lisa chose her fear over her mother's loving concern. A few years later when Lisa was at a summer camp a boy sneaked into her cabin to scare the girls. She significantly over reacted, cowering in the corner and not sleeping the rest of the night. The next day she insisted on going home, and became defiant of the rules until she was sent home. Her counselor recognized that this event had been significant and what it might represent so carefully asked her about her home life or events that might have prompted her response. Even though her uncle moved away and was out of the picture at this time, Lisa refused to say anything.

 The older Lisa became the more defiant her behavior became because of the dissonance within her body. She was trying to pretend all was well and had suppressed her memories but the subconscious was trying to be heard. That is when the drinking had begun. She was able to hide it from her parents for a time, however eventually they became aware of it. Finally, during college when she was taken to the emergency room due to a lethal amount of alcohol in her system, they stepped in. She went into rehab and counseling. This worked fairly well for Lisa but mostly because it scared her enough to make her change her behavior, not because she recognized her own worth and the love of her parents. So the fear only motivated her for a period of time. The lessons still needed to be learned.

However, it was during this time of fear-based behavior that she met and fell in love with Wes. Again, God put someone in her path that could help her learn to trust and love herself. Wes did truly love Lisa. But as we all know, love does not cure all things. Because of Wes' own patterns and misunderstandings of his way of communicating this love, Lisa went back into her old patterns of thinking and eventually drinking to cover up the pain.

At this point in Lisa's life she had convinced herself to believe the story she had created for herself over the years. She believed that she was not worthy of love, that her only value was her physical beauty. Therefore, when that went, no one would ever want her. She believed she wasn't a strong enough person to ever be able to overcome her drinking. Lisa, like all of us, was heavily invested in her story because she had spent a lifetime creating it. Debbie Ford talks about this concept also in her book *The Dark Side of The Light Chasers*, "The power you need is there, but it will only come out when your desire to change your life is stronger than your desire to stay the same. When we lose touch with ourselves we lose touch with our divinity, and because we don't trust ourselves, we come to believe that other people can't be trusted." To admit our story may not be correct or to abandon it would be akin to committing suicide. After all, who would Lisa be, or who would any of us be, if we aren't who we have supposed ourselves to be all these years?

When trauma has been experienced by my clients and they feel it was done intentionally by another person, like Lisa or even Lindsay back in chapter 8, the client gives away one of their most precious aspects of themselves to those they detest and those they love without even knowing it. This is their aspect of humanness. The aspect of being imperfect, of realizing so much of what we don't like in others is the same thing we don't like about ourselves.....the vulnerability. They become, over time, someone created by suppressed emotions and trying desperately to fit into whatever mold they have created for themselves rather than accepting circumstances as gifts so they can become the brilliant, creative, divine person they were meant to be in this existence.

Lisa, like each of us, had to find the courage to rediscover who she truly could be and was in reality. She had to accept that God was there for her, guiding her and blessing her with opportunities to heal and recognize the beautiful and lovable person she had been created to be. By examining her life from this perspective and recognizing the people he had put in her path, she was able to see the gifts God had tried to give her and was once again offering her.

She was able to understand the role her uncle played in her theatrical production of life. That was all it was, a role, played by another human being. That understanding gave her empowerment to see the role she also played and disassociate from the shame she had linked with the events. Once understanding and disassociation happened so did forgiveness. With the forgiveness came acceptance and

133

self-love. With acceptance and self-love came the greatest gift, the gift to *heal thyself*.

Chapter 10

How To Find A Practitioner

"But the genius of this work is simply the magic of what happens between the two—the client and the healer."

~ Hugh Milne, DO, *The Heart of Listening: A Visionary Approach to Cranio- Sacral Therapy*

So far I've introduced you to the history and the theory of craniosacral therapy. I've walked you through several case studies so you could hopefully relate to how it works. So in the next couple of chapters I want to prepare you to know how to have an rewarding experience if you decide craniosacral therapy is for you.

As important and effective as craniosacral therapy is, it is **just as important** to select a therapist that is right for you. Dr. Hugh Milne also comments in his book that, "The client is oriented to the therapist, not a therapy."

He adds, and I fully agree, that you need to find someone who honors the stillness of the work, as well as the understanding that what needs to happen, will happen if he/she can simply create an open, non-directive environment. A gifted practitioner is someone who believes wholeheartedly that when given an open space, the human body and the soul's wisdom will figure out what is best for the body and the soul together.

Finding this practitioner can take some effort on the client's part. There is a list of practitioners on The Upledger Institute's website, www.Upledger.com. However, you will see, as I mentioned earlier, that there are several people who have studied the first course of Craniosacral Therapy (CST I) and considerably less that have taken CST II or above. This list is a good starting point though. There is also a practitioner list on Biodynamic Craniosacral Therapy Association's website, www.craniosacraltherapy.org. Although Biodynamic's approach is slightly different that Upledger's the therapy achieves the same results. This is what Dr. Milne meant about the client not being oriented to the specific approach but to the therapist doing the therapy.

Once you have found a few practitioners in your geographical area that have had more than the first level of studies and training, it is time to make some telephone calls. The following is a list of questions I would suggest you discuss with the practitioner before deciding to schedule an appointment with them. If a practitioner is not willing to take the time to answer all of your questions to your satisfaction move on to the next one, until you find one who will.

Also, if you are the type of person who is hesitant to ask a professional these types of questions, you will need to get over that reluctance. This is your health, your life and your money. It is an investment in your life and choosing the right practitioner who is going to direct your healing process requires as much time and effort as you would put into any other major investment.

Here are important questions to ask:

- **How long have you been doing Craniosacral Therapy (CST)?** Although this can't be your only deciding factor, experience does count. Remember my story of the orthodontist that got me into this work? He told me to give it ten years or so. However, there is one thing to be said about someone new to the work and that is that often they are more open to the body directing the session simply because they don't have the experience of where a session of a specific situation "usually" goes.

- **How much of your professional time is spent doing CST versus other forms of therapy?**

  Most practitioners whether massage therapists, physical therapists, chiropractors, doctors or nurses that do CST have come to it secondarily in their career path. Make sure CST is a large part of their everyday client base. Otherwise you run the risk of the CST being a diluted form or offshoot of their primary therapy.

- **Why do you personally do CST?**

  The way that a practitioner answers this question will give you insight to their feelings about CST but also their personality and approach. One thing you want to be looking for is that the practitioner believes the therapy does the work or that each situation is different because the therapy is individual to the client.

- **What is CST?**

Why ask this question when you have already read this book and have a pretty good understanding of the therapy? Because you want to make sure your practitioner knows the therapy well enough to be able to explain it in terms you can understand. It will help you know they are significantly acquainted with the therapy but it will also help you know if this is someone you can communicate with comfortably and accurately. This is a critical aspect of a client/practitioner relationship.

- **What types of situations do you personally have experience treating?**

It is nice if you can find someone who has experience with what you are dealing with but, because of the far reaching healing effects of CST, it isn't crucial. One thing you don't want to hear in response to this question is, "pretty much everything". I don't know a practitioner out there who can honestly make this statement. Sometimes it feels that way but if they are being honest and humble with you they will be specific. And for this therapy, honest and humble are critical traits.

- **What is your experience with (insert your condition or concerns)?**

    You might find the answer to this question in the practitioner's response to the preceding question. But if not, then be sure to bring up your situation and pay attention again to their response. It should be sincere and specific. Generalized answers, such as, "oh yes, I've dealt with that" isn't an adequate response that says you and your condition are important.

- **How many sessions are required for my condition or concern?**

    There is no right or wrong answer here except, "it could take a year or more". CST will be beneficial to you or it won't. I ask my clients to commit to three one hour sessions with no more than a week between sessions. At the end of those three sessions both you and I should have an idea if cranial therapy is helping you enough to continue with additional sessions. **NOTE**: this does not mean you will be healed in three sessions! It means you will notice enough of a difference in pain levels, sleep patterns, anxiety levels or whatever it is we are working on, that you and I will want to persist in our healing relationship. Also, I think it is important that your practitioner convey to you their confidence, not only in the therapy, but in your body. What I mean is that I don't want you or your body to become dependant on the therapist or the therapy. That isn't healing. So after an initial set of sessions, perhaps three or six or even eight (probably not more than that) I encourage my clients to start extending the time between sessions to see what their bodies will do. This gives you and your new body a chance to continue to adapt and heal using its own intellect.

Please keep in mind when considering healing time that it probably took several months or even years to get your body where it is when you start craniosacral therapy. It will be a process to achieve wellness again.

- **How will I know if the therapy is working?**

We all seem to have some kind of expectations. I have worked hard on letting go of expectations but still fall into old patterns at times. I find it important to find out what my clients expectations are so we can discuss them and eventually agree on a treatment expectation for our three sessions. However, I feel it is important for you as the client to see what your practitioner's expectations of your sessions are. This question will help open the door for that discussion to take place. If the practitioner's response to this question is too vague for you pursue a more clearly defined answer. But, be sure to know what your expectations are too.

Sometimes the results are extremely profound and obvious. Other times they are subtle and not as obvious to a person unfamiliar with this type of therapy.

I personally have found it very helpful to have my clients fill out a symptom form before we begin our first session, which lists numerous symptoms and gives the client the opportunity to rate their response on a scale from 0 to 5. 0 represents *never* and 5 characterizes *most the time* or *severe*. I then ask them to fill it out again at the end of the three sessions without giving them back their first copy. When they have finished completing the form the second time we sit and compare the responses. This way both the client and I can see where they have improved. I know it sounds odd but over and over again, I've observed that *once a person is feeling better; they forget how bad they felt.* This selective memory is one of the coping mechanisms of our brain. For instance, if you are a woman who has gone through childbirth, and you could actually remember in full detail that excruciating pain, would you do it again?

- **Do I still need to take my medications or continue with my traditional medical care?**

  The only practitioner who can take you off medications or recommend you discontinue a medical protocol, is a medical doctor. Other practitioners such as an acupuncturist, a chiropractor, a nurse or physical therapist, even a nutritionist or massage therapist can suggest you discuss a certain medication or protocol with your doctor because of a specific concern or recommendation they have. But it is only a recommendation. If anyone tells you to stop a medication or protocol prescribed by your physician because craniosacral therapy will cure you, proceed with great caution.

- **Do you work in the mouth? How often?**

  As I've mentioned before most practitioners have come to CST as a secondary therapy to their primary licensing therapy. Because of this many, other than dentists, are uncomfortable putting their hands in a person's mouth. I've encountered many practitioners who have had multiple levels of training, including the mouth work, who are not including it in their regular protocols or sessions. They just aren't at ease with it. But **mouth work** is an absolute critical part of the therapy, in my opinion. Too many of the bones and tissues of the mouth attach to the rest of the skull and a practitioner is not doing full justice to the therapy or the client if they are not doing mouth work.

- **Do you have a website I can review?**

  Again, this is not a "must have" but if they do have one perusing it can often give you a good feeling for the approach a therapist takes, their background, and their knowledge and experience. Also, ask them if they provided the writing for it or if they had it professionally done. If they did the writing themselves it will give you an idea of their ability to communicate and if you can easily follow their thinking and reasoning process.

A Practitioner Who Supports A Healthy Lifestyle

As for myself, I feel it is also vital to look at the client's lifestyle because their daily life can have a significant impact on their health condition and on how effective my therapy is going to be for them. Therefore I have a health history interview with my clients that will give me insights to the whole person. Keep in mind a practitioner who is exceptional in their craft can't do it all, so I appreciate those practitioners who have a network of colleagues they can acquaint you with that will aid in your overall healing process. Some practitioners I know do wonderful CST but aren't comfortable with the Emotional Release Therapy. So when they come up to a blockage that requires this particular therapy they have someone else for their clients to see.

Nutritional intake when trying to heal is fundamental to achieving wellness goals. Hormonal issues play a huge part in the body being able to hold the cranial or chiropractic adjustments clients are receiving. Movement is paramount to healing. Movement can mean running to walking, to dancing, to bowling. Having a network of talented teachers and practitioners who your practitioner can refer you to is always a bonus worth looking for in your healer. Not only because it makes your life richer and easier but because it shows that your practitioner sees the wholeness of the healing process and will be there with you through the entire journey.

Another really wonderful way to find a gifted practitioner is to ask friends and contacts. A good referral speaks volumes about a practitioner. Even if you can only get a referral for a great chiropractor or physical therapist, they often times will know someone who does CST.

A Google search will sometimes help but be sure to approach the responses the same as the data bases mentioned previously and ask your questions.

You And Your Intuition

But most of all... trust your intuition. As I've discussed in the previous chapters, a portion of the healing process of craniosacral therapy is about re-claiming your primary emotions and yourself. Please believe that your body knows better than me or anyone else what it needs. Once you've done your research and spoke to different practitioners then find a quiet place to "be with the information." Don't analyze or judge it, just allow it to soak in. Then when one name becomes more prevalent in your thoughts, trust your body and schedule the appointment.

Along this same line, I would encourage you to trust your intuition and your body as therapy is progressing. In a quality professional relationship between a practitioner and a client there needs to be an environment for open and honest communication. If you find that during a session you feel any thought or idea is being pushed on you or that what is coming up for discussion just doesn't feel right then you need to be able to comfortably express that discomfort or misfit.

For instance, when I am trying to help a client recognize a behavior pattern or a possible misguided emotion I paraphrase my comments with, "How does it feel to you if I say, I think it might be….anger. Does that ring true for you?" Or if I think their lifestyle choice of being in a career that is totally stressing them out needs looked at I might say, "What do you think is the worst thing that would happen if you chose to leave that job?" In other words, it can't be the practitioner's session, it must be your session and the information and work must ring true to what resonate with your body. The craniosacral rhythm will help the therapist stay on track if you're avoiding the subject versus it not feeling correct to you.

I've had people call me who "don't want to hurt their therapist's feelings" but don't feel like they are getting anywhere or are getting uncomfortable with the sessions. A truly professional therapist or practitioner will be more concerned about their client's comfort and progress than their business. There have been times when I have reached a plateau with one of my clients, referred them to a colleague, and they have started progressing again. I can not emphasize enough that it is the synergy of client and practitioner that creates the open space for the body to heal. A quality practitioner will understand this and applaud you for acknowledging it also. If for any reason the practitioner tries to make you feel guilty about changing, first take a step back and ask if he/she is really laying a guilt trip on you or whether because of your history, you are choosing to feel guilty. Then trust your original instincts and move on to someone else. But, if in your self-evaluation you realized it was more you choosing guilt then bring that up with your new practitioner so the source of that choice can be examined.

YOU *ARE* AN EQUAL

Also, you should be able to feel as though you are an equal in your healing process. If you find that during your sessions you feel as though the practitioner is not fully present with you or that they are not listening to your concerns or awareness, it is probably time to find a different practitioner. This is another aspect of building a trust with your body and intuition as well as with your practitioner.

Dr. Andrew Still, the father of osteopathy, said, "Anyone can find disease, but how do we find health? We can not cure anything with Craniosacral Therapy. We simply facilitate the patient's self-healing."

Dr. John Upledger added to this sentiment, "The shortest distance between two points is [a healing] intention."

Find a practitioner **who** is humble enough to embody these two statements, who believes in your body and has the intention to empower it with health.

Then you will be in excellent... and healing... hands.

Chapter 11

How To Get The Most Out Of Craniosacral Therapy

As I began the rough draft of this chapter I found myself thinking that the suggestions I was making for enhancing your therapy are too lengthy and could be overwhelming for any person, but particularly for those of you who are experiencing debilitating pain or exhaustion due to illness or emotional issues. So I decided I would list the top three areas of concern and suggest you work on those first and then others as you feel you are capable. However, on approximately the sixth revision of the top three in importance I decided it couldn't be done.

As a therapist I see all the suggestions as critical steps in creating wellness as well as wholeness for my clients. So I suggest you simply read through this chapter knowing that when you take your first steps down this path you will remember it is a journey, and not a short one either. But once you have started traversing the path you will find some slopes fairly easy to climb while others will require starts and stops along the way.

Try taking these enhancement suggestions one at a time. Each week that you are progressing with your therapy discuss with your therapist which one(s) you should focus on for that week. Overtime, you will find that they are no longer suggestions you have to work at, but merely healthy lifestyle habits you have created as part of your wellness routine.

To help make this information more easily digestible I've divided the information into two chapters; physical (body) and emotional (spirit). However, as you have hopefully noticed throughout this book my mantra is that the mind and the body cannot be separated but need to be treated as one entity. Therefore, try to work on one item from each chapter as you progress.

Healing The Body Suggestions

Hydration

Your body depends on water for survival. Water makes up more than two thirds of your body weight. Every cell, tissue and organ in your body needs water to function correctly. For example, your body uses water to maintain its temperature, remove waste and lubricate joints. Therefore, when you are trying to make changes in the tissues and the cells with therapy you need to be giving the body enough fluid that it can actually make the changes necessary.

148

Amazingly, many of the symptoms that people come into my office for treating are identical to those people are suffering from dehydration, namely, headaches, fatigue, dizziness, joint pain, muscular pain, mental fatigue or forgetfulness and depression. This is not to say that all of these will simply disappear from your life if you drink more water, but it is difficult to resolve these issues if on top of the craniosacral issues, you are working against yourself by not hydrating the tissues and cells so that the dehydration exacerbates the symptoms.

As your therapist works to release tensed muscles, release scar tissue and myofasical restrictions in the soft tissue this will release toxins that have been stored in these tissues. Without adequate water to flush these toxins out of your system through the kidneys, liver or perspiration you can end up experiencing the same symptoms listed in the paragraph above. In fact it is almost certain you will feel worse the day after your session than when you came in for treatment.

Different people need different amounts of water. On About.com the nutritional web pages have a calculator you can use to determine how much water you need according to your specific situation. You can find the calculator at http://nutrition.about.com/library/blwatercalculator.htm.
However, a good rule of thumb for how much water to consume is to take your body weight in pounds and divide it in half. Then try to consume at least that amount of ounces in non-caffeinated and non-alcoholic drinks per day. So if your weight is 150 pounds you would divide that in half equaling 75 pounds. Now convert that to 75 ounces and that is your daily goal. This does not reflect the water or liquid used for cooking or meal planning, but simply the liquids you drink each day. It also does not include the amount of additional fluid you need if you are exercising heavily.

It is important to keep in mind that caffeinated and alcoholic drinks have a dehydrating effect on the body. Therefore, you need to minimize the amounts of these types of drinks you consume or you will need to increase your intake of water above the formulated amount. Also, please keep in mind that fruit juices and soda have large amounts of sugar in them and therefore should be used sparingly.

The best source of hydration is filtered water. Because many sources of tap water and bottled water have high doses of toxins in them, you are better off purchasing and installing a filter system in your home. If you get tired of plain filtered water, add a slice of lemon, lime or cucumber for a refreshing alternative.

Sleep

If you will remember in Lisa's case study, she talked about how tired she was at the end of the sessions. This is due in part to the emotional issues being dealt with but also because as the body makes tissue changes it requires the body to burn energy to make the changes. The body will require adequate sleep to be able to generate the usable energy it needs to make the changes and shifts necessary for the body to maintain the new structure.

I recommend to my clients that they plan a restful evening the day of their sessions. If given the chance the body will tell you it needs rest and relaxation to complete whatever it is working on after a session. Often times clients tell me that they have slept 10-12 hours the night after their first session. This is because the body's nervous system has been under enormous stress for a period of time, and now has been given permission to relax. Do yourself a favor and allow your body the time to sleep if it wants it.

According to several sources an average of 30% of the American population suffers from insomnia during a 12 month period of time. Sources also state that we are sleeping 20% less now than Americans did 100 years ago. And yet sleep is an important part of a healthy body. Sleep regulates the release of important hormones, slows the aging process, boosts immune system function, as well as brain function and reduces cortisol levels which decreases our ability to deal with stress, creates irritability and anxiety.

A good solid night's sleep restores, repairs and replenishes your body. Here are a few important questions to ask yourself.

- Do you need an alarm clock to wake up?
- Do you feel drowsy driving short distances or waiting at traffic lights?
- Do you feel sleepy and have a difficult time focusing mid-afternoon?
- Do you get irritable or agitated easily? (Ask a family member or co-worker this question.)
- Do you wake up easily with every noise in the night?
- Are you a chronic worrier?

If you answer yes to any of these, most likely you aren't getting enough sleep. Therefore, you are doing yourself and your health a disservice. If you are having difficulty sleeping try a couple of these easy fixes. Go to bed by 10:00 PM. The body's internal clock starts turning "on" some organ functions at 10:00 PM and if you are not going to sleep when that process begins, you will most likely get a second wind and start waking up again. Also avoid all caffeine and refined sugars after 2 PM. Don't watch high action movies or TV before going to bed. Let your mind start to calm down for the hour before bedtime.

If you find these simple suggestions, when followed for a period of time, do not work for you then you may want to consider natural sleep aids. I would recommend seeing a holistic health care practitioner if your insomnia is severe, but you could safely try taking Valerian Root which is a sedative herb used to induce relaxation and therefore sleep. It can be brewed as a tea but I find it easier to take by capsule form. You can take 300 - 600 mg about an hour before bedtime. If you are already taking a prescription medication for insomnia be sure to discuss the addition of Valerian Root with your doctor.

Other natural solutions might be 5 HTP which is an amino acid which helps raise serotonin levels to encourage sleep. A usual dose would be 150 – 300 mg daily an hour before bedtime or if that doesn't work try 100 mg two hours before bedtime and another 100 mg again an hour before bedtime. According to "Alternative and Integral Therapies for Insomnia" calcium and magnesium are important minerals needed by the body for many functions, one of which is sleep. Magnesium citrate is a natural muscle relaxant. Therefore, if generalized muscle or body pain is keeping you awake, try taking 200 – 400 mg nightly. This article also references melatonin which is a hormone the body produces to help our bodies sleep. It will only help if you are actually low in your production of melatonin naturally in your body. Lack of light is what causes our body to produce melatonin. So make sure your bedroom is dark. Start shutting down bright lights, especially computer and telephone screens about an hour before bedtime.

Movement

The body's most important nutrient is oxygen. We can go weeks without food, a day or two without water but only minutes without oxygen. It is an absolute requirement of our bodies. Aerobic exercise, or movement, means "with air". What better way to give our bodies the much needed oxygen than movement with air?

When our bodies are deprived of oxygen they suffer from fatigue, memory loss, sleep disorders, depression, lowered libido, joint and muscle pain, infections, and blood sugar regulation problems. They also have trouble absorbing and metabolizing fats. Does this list sound familiar? It is very similar to the list for dehydration and for those suffering with chronic pain and illness.

The primary purpose of the lymphatic system of the body is to carry away toxins therefore detoxifying the body, helping to keep it healthy. It is a system of capillaries and vessels all over the body and organs with small vents that open and close pushing the fluid through the system, to the lymph nodes cleansing the fluid and re-dispensing it back into the body. This system is driven by the muscular system of the body rather than the cardiovascular system. Without proper movement of the muscles of the body this system becomes stagnant allowing the toxins in the body to build up.

You do not need to run marathons or power lift weights to accomplish the healing power of movement. The National Cancer Institute published an article "Cancer Trends Progress Report – 2005 Update." It stated "increasing physical activity at work or during leisure time to include walking briskly 30 minutes a day could lower the risk of getting colon cancer by 50%". The Journal of American Medical Association found that women who engaged in the same amount of exercise (30 minutes a day) decreased their chances of breast cancer by 18 percent.

Moderate exercise has also been shown to increase heart function making a person less likely to suffer from hypertensive diseases, lower blood pressure, reduce body fat, increase bone mass, enhance and balance hormone levels, eliminate toxins from the body, strengthen muscles and tendons, as well as increase brain function.

These are the wonderful physical benefits of exercise, but just as important are the emotional benefits of moving the body. I've witnessed many of my clients report feeling better about their appearance, having an improved self-image and greater self-confidence primarily because they are taking control of how their body looks and feels through exercise.

David Klein, Ph.D., Hygienic MD, in *Living Nutrition* has this to say about exercise. "Exercise unites the mind, body, and spirit by activating will power, motivation, desire, self-reliance, and self-awareness. Gaining coordination over one's thoughts, emotions, and body generates a rewarding sense of self-satisfaction, capability, and physical and mental strength. Mindfulness becomes an overall coping mechanism for successful recovery and healing."

Typically when someone says the word *exercise*, people think of runners, trekking off to a gym, or lifting heavy weights. But keep an open mind here. Think of brisk walking, cycling, and swimming, dancing, skating, skiing, golfing (if you walk) or maybe even playing basketball. Building muscle is an important part of exercising so using weights is important but using your body weight to accomplish certain exercises is just as effective as purchasing weights or going to a gym. This is one of the reasons I love yoga. It not only stretches the muscles and tissues but it helps build strength as well. Generally speaking, unless doing power yoga, it is an exercise that moves slowly from one movement to another helping you become reacquainted with your body. It also promotes breathing which improves the oxygen flow to your muscles and your brain. Other considerations are Thi Chi and Pilates.

The key is to find something you enjoy doing, sticking with it and having fun. Of course it helps if you have an exercise buddy for those days you just don't feel like getting out there yourself. They can encourage you. Also important is to mix things up; don't just do the same thing, at the same place over and over again. You will get bored with the routine of it and your body will become too conditioned so that the exercise will not be as effective for you as it was when you started.

Nutrition

I have left this subject until last, not because it is the least important, but because I feel it is such a vast subject with the largest amount of confusion and therefore pitfalls. What we hear is safe and good for us to eat one month will often be deemed unhealthy in the near future. At one point we will be told we should eat a high protein, low carbohydrate diet and later be told too much protein in the diet isn't good for us.

Also my experience with many people is that they are emotionally attached to food more than almost anything else in their life, barring a chemical addiction. When you think about it food is a mainstay of our social world. When was the last time you attended a social event, whether it was a movie, a party, a sporting event, or even a hike with friends that food wasn't a part of it? To make it even more challenging most of the time the food offerings at these events aren't the healthiest choice for our bodies.

Yet our nutritional intake from the food we eat is critically important when it comes to how our bodies heal and function. I don't suppose any of you would spend $200,000.00 on a new Ferrari sports coupe only to put the cheapest leaded fuel in it, would you? But how much thought do we put into putting processed, genetically altered food into our priceless human engines?

I would like to make five suggestions that my clients have told me were helpful in raising their awareness of nutritional intake.

First it is important to know what types of food your personal body works best with. Dr. Joseph Mercola gives a wealth of knowledge on his website and in his newsletters. He tends to be a little too dogmatic for my personal approach but one concept of his I really appreciate and encourage my clients to do, is to take his nutritional typing test. It is free and gives you insight to whether you will do best with proteins, carbohydrates, fats, or a combination of any two. He also provides a week's worth of menu planning for your meals to give you an idea of what your intake would realistically look like on a given day if you follow the typing. You can find this test at http://nutritionaltyping.mercola.com/login.aspx.

Once you know what types of foods you are going to help you function the most optimally eating, it is time to go grocery shopping. This is where many people get sabotaged. Food companies know how to market and label their foods to make them appealing and salable. My second recommendation is to stay on the perimeter of the grocery store. When you enter a grocery store, most of the time, the fresh produce is set up on one side of the store, the meat department on the back, and the dairy and bakery sections on the other side. That is where you want to do the majority of your shopping. Once you get into the middle of the store you are dealing with processed foods.

The third concept I ask clients to consider is purchasing organic. I have had mixed feelings about this for years. For one thing it is more expensive and secondly the government controls for what determines organic are under monitored. However, the more toxic our environment has become the more important I feel it is to reduce exposure every way we can. A good way to do this in the summer is to buy locally. There are often times places you can go and even pick your own produce so you get not only pesticide free but freshly picked instead of picked green and held for months in storage. According to the Environmental Working Group an organization of scientists, researchers and policy makers, certain types of organic produce can reduce your exposure to toxic chemicals by as much as 80%. Perhaps you have heard of the "Dirty Dozen" and the "Clean 15". These different fruits and vegetables listed on the dirty dozen tested positive to having anywhere from 47-65 toxic chemicals in them when grown conventionally. The clean 15 tested negative to most chemicals.

"Dirty Dozen"

- celery
- peaches
- strawberries
- apples
- domestic blueberries
- nectarines
- sweet bell peppers
- spinach, kale and collard greens
- cherries
- potatoes
- imported grapes
- lettuce

"Clean 15"

- onions
- avocados
- sweet corn
- pineapples
- mango
- sweet peas
- asparagus
- kiwi fruit
- cabbage
- eggplant
- cantaloupe
- watermelon
- grapefruit
- sweet potatoes
- sweet onions

The other idea to explore along the lines of organic is the meat you choose. Grass fed without antibiotics and hormones is definitely a healthier choice. US Wellness Meats tells us we are paying in other ways besides the antibiotics and hormones though. "…one need only look to our beef-loving neighbors in Argentina to understand how. Though Argentina leads the world in per-capita red meat consumption, the country enjoys lower numbers in deaths-per-1000 of heart disease, diabetes and cancer. And, yes, Argentina has specialized in grass-fed beef production for centuries."

Time magazine published an article in their June 2006 magazine detailing the movement of turning from high volume, antibiotic, hormone driven meat industry to what one reformed rancher calls, "tuning in to real food";
http:/www.time.com/time/magazine/article/0.9171.1200759.00.html#izz1VV5dPYg.

If you are feeling indecisive about going organic, perhaps you can start with these three areas, the "Dirty Dozen", the

"Clean 15" and grass fed meat and dairy. Just making those changes could make a big difference in your health.

The fourth suggestion is tracking and planning your nutritional intake. When I ask my clients to keep a food journal for just a week and to include not only what they ate and how much but to include in it how they felt an hour or two after eating they often put up resistance. For one thing, none of us want one more thing to do in our already hectic daily life. But this is a crucial step to wellness. It serves a very important purpose; **awareness.**

Due to our busy hectic schedules we often don't pay attention to what we actually eat, how often or how much. It is just something we do and that can be a pitfall. But by actually documenting what you ate, and when and how much, even for just one week, you will become mindful of the fuel you are putting into your engine. You will also become aware in part as to why you are feeling the way you are and how it relates to your nutritional intake.

After keeping track of this information for a week sit down at your computer or grab a reference guide and start evaluating what you have asked your body to process over the last week. Look up calories and look up the grams of carbohydrates relative to grams of protein...ideally they should be in a 3/1 ration carbs/proteins. Also notice grams of fat and sugar. To lose weight Dr. Joseph Mercola states you should keep your total sugar grams to 15-16 grams a day and to maintain under 20 grams a day. You will find that most standard American diets have three and four times that much. If your blood sugar levels are constantly up and down it will be difficult to feel good and make the changes your body wants to make while going through your craniosacral therapy sessions.

The fifth proposal I make for clients is to consider portion control. A couple of years ago I had the delightful experience of visiting Thailand. One of the remarkable observations I made while there, was that I didn't see any obese people. More importantly was the fact that the people I did see, and there were plenty of them in Bangkok, had vibrant skin, silky shining hair and focused clear eyes. I commented to my host about this and his response was, "well look at what they eat; lots of fish, fresh foods, very little dairy or wheat and lots of rice." The only fast food establishment I saw while there was McDonalds. Although I didn't want to eat McDonalds I wanted to go in one to see how they differed from the ones here in the States. The menu was similar but there were no large sizes and definitely not the option to "super size" any order. The hamburgers and French fries orders were small in comparison and the drink cups were one size; small. I remember thinking Americans probably wouldn't put up with this and would just move on to a competitor who would "super size" their order.

But even when you are trying to be conscious about what and how much you are eating it is often difficult to determine what is considered a healthy serving of a particular food. I've put together a quick reference list of portion control that I give my clients. A more extensive list that can be printed to fit in a wallet or put on the refrigerator can be seen at http:/webmed.com/diet/printable/wallet-portion-control-size-guide.

Rice or Pasta	Size of a 60 watt light bulb
Baked Potato	Size of computer mouse
Bagel (half)	Size of a hockey puck
Muffin	Size of a large egg
Meats	Size of your palm (size & thickness)
Nuts	Size of a ping-pong ball

Butter	Size of the tip of your thumb
Cheese	Size of two dice
Raw veggies	Size of your fist (1 cup)
Cooked veggies	Size of a 60 watt light bulb
Fruit	Size of a tennis ball

By using these five suggestions you can improve your nutritional intake significantly. Once you have mastered these suggestions you may feel like taking even more control over your eating habits. At that time there are numerous books written on the subject. Almost too many, in that it can be an overwhelming task to find what works for you. But that is the key. You need to find what style of eating healthy you can make yours and your family's lifestyle. The key is to realize it isn't a diet, it isn't about losing weight it is all about lifestyle and getting and staying healthy so you can take pleasure in your life.

Chapter 12

How To Get The Most Out Of Craniosacral Therapy (Part II)

As I stated in the previous chapter, the suggestions found there and the ones identified here are both equally important to the overall healing process. However, most people will tend to minimize the suggestions in this chapter partially because they are not linear in fashion.

The human mind likes linear thinking. There is a time line, first we do this and next we do that and end with this. It is simple and it makes sense. Conversely when we are dealing with the spirit and emotions they are not linear and often times are difficult to get our brains around.

For this reason I believe this is the chapter that many of the readers will either blow off as unimportant or they will not

162

read at all. Or they will look at the heading and say "I will deal with this later." **Well later has arrived**.

I have had clients tell me that they don't believe in meditation. It doesn't fit into their religious belief system. They have expressed concerns of evil spirits trying to influence their minds or of being "brainwashed". To those people I ask them if they believe that through prayer God can bless them, then why would he not protect them and guide them through focused quiet time? We are responsible for our thoughts since they obviously precede our actions. If necessary you can start your meditation/quiet time with a prayer asking God to guide your meditation time and protect you from evil thoughts. You are in control of your thoughts.

Of course there is always the objection that people don't have time. But we all know that is simply an excuse. We all have the same amount of time and how we choose to use it is critical to our well-being. I discuss this at much greater length below in the section on **Stress**.

So please, once again, I'm asking you to open your mind and your heart to the possibilities of finding a new healthier you.

Healing the Spirit Suggestions

Writing or Journaling

Years ago I read Julia Cameron's book "The Artist's Way". In this book she encourages people to do "Morning Pages" in order to unblock and free their creative self. As I read the book and started doing the exercises, I found them helpful for discovering more than my creative self....I found myself.

Then as I started doing the emotional release therapy with my clients I found we were unveiling aspects of their lives and themselves that were new to them and that this knowledge was useful, but often, even though the body cleared the memory, the client's brain now wanted to process it somehow. I started using a variation of Ms. Cameron's *Morning Pages* to help my clients. From the session, we would come up with a question or statement that they needed to process. They would write the question as an open unfinished statement allowing their intuition to write the ending.

Let me share an example with you. Remember Lindsay, whose husband constantly blamed her for his unfaithfulness and indiscretions back in chapter 8? She had very low self esteem and felt there wasn't anything she could do right or well. Even though we found the source of this belief and processed it from her tissues it was difficult for her brain to accept the truth after believing the lie for so long. So Lindsay started her *Morning Writings*. She would sit each and every day and begin her writing with "What I need to feel loveable is...."

These writing assignments that I give my clients have only three rules. They are:

1. Get rid of distractions. No phones, noise or other people around.
2. Set the timer for 5 minutes. Once you start the timer your pen touches the paper and it doesn't come off the paper until the timer goes off. Of course if you are writing something and information is flowing when the timer goes off, you can gladly continue writing for as long as your heart desires. The five minutes is a minimum.
3. Don't go back and read what you wrote.

You can probably understand the reasoning and importance of rule number one. So I will go on to explain the other two rules. The first thing most clients say is "But I won't know what to write for five minutes. I don't know how to finish that statement." They are correct; they probably won't be able to finish the statement...at first. So they continue to write the part that is given to them over and over until either the timer goes off or they think of something else to write at the end of the statement.

You and your body know the ending to the statement. But that information has been buried for quite a while. Your body isn't sure if it can totally trust you that if it gives you the information you will do anything with it or even worse, fears you will dismiss the information as unimportant. Therefore, it takes time to coax the information from within. It may take a few minute of writing or rewriting the unfinished statement as is before some ending starts to come forth. Or it may take several days. Just stick with the process. It is worth it in the end.

The third rule, it is important not go back and read what you wrote. Your critical survival self has learned coping mechanisms that have, layer by layer covered up and muddied over what your subconscious is trying to get you to recognize and accept. If you go back and read what you wrote, your critical self will start to diminish what you have written and maybe even justify why you've ignored this part of yourself. As Ingrid Bengis said, 'Words are a form of action, capable of influencing change." Simply getting the words out of the brain and onto the paper will spur you on to the change that is needed to move forward. I've seen it over and over again.

For those of you who are reading this book and looking for improvements or who are working with another therapist and want to make the most of your sessions, start writing. It doesn't really matter if you have the jump start of the theme your subconscious is trying to convey to you. With or without the theme the message will eventually come through your free flow writing. Make a commitment to write for even just 5 minutes a day. Do it every day without going back and reading it. Write whatever is going through your mind, even if it is your "to do" list for the day. Eventually, other insights will begin to come through and changes will begin to happen.

Meditation/Quiet Time

Meditation or having quiet time is similar to writing. It is giving our inner self permission to express itself and make known to our conscious self details we need to know. Often people shy away from the mention of meditation because they immediately have visions of monks sitting on hard floors for long periods of time or hippies on pillows, chanting over and over while incense is burning. If that is where your mind is going, it is time to change the channel and open your mind to a different reality. Meditation has become mainstream. Corporate management consultants, in pursuit of physical and mental health have learned to think of meditation primarily as a stress-management tool. Spiritual seekers choose to view meditation as a gateway to God or divine inspiration. Artists and creative muses endorse it as a conduit for greater creativity. These approaches are all correct but there is a purpose much greater about meditation. Again I quote from *The Artist's Way,* "We meditate to discover our own identity, our right place in the scheme of the universe. Through meditation, we acquire and eventually acknowledge our connection to an inner power source that has the ability to transform our outer world. In other words, meditation gives us not only the light of insight but also the power for expansive change."

Remember that your body knows everything and has everything it needs to heal, when given the proper environment. Meditation gives us the tool to know what it is our body needs in order to create the proper environment whether it be emotional, physical, spiritual or any combination.

One of the main blessings meditation gives to your body is the ability to be in the present moment. When we are in the present moment we can simply *be*. We don't have to worry about the past or concern ourselves with the future. We don't have to long for when we get that next promotion, when the children are grown, when I am healthy again, when I have/had more energy...we are simply observing *what is*.

Many of my clients say that they can't quiet their brain. It just keeps chattering away at them. I have to smile at this comment because I remember when I was where they are now. I remember reading books on meditation that would say to empty your mind or to simply focus on your breath. But my mind wouldn't stay empty or stay focused on my boring breath. Then one beautiful spring day I was setting on my front porch just taking a breather from the craziness inside my house when a car came driving up the street. The neighbor's dog was outside and when the dog saw the car he immediately started chasing the car. He continued for a short time and then gave up and ambled back to his shady place under the tree. Only a few minutes later another car came around the corner and started up our street. Again, the dog's ears perked up and off it went in pursuit of this new car only to give up and amble back and relax. I thought to myself what a senseless waist of time and energy these pursuits were for this dog. But obviously the pattern served some sort of purpose beyond my understanding.

Then I had an "aha" moment. Weren't the thoughts that passed through my brain when I was trying to empty my brain very similar to the dog chasing the car? The thought comes, hangs around for a moment and then is gone and I return to my peacefulness. I didn't need to understand or process the thought I simply needed to let it pass through and then return to rest in my favorite shady spot. The process of chasing cars or emptying my mind no longer needed to make sense to me. I could merely allow it.

When I was able to let go of the effort of emptying my mind or focusing on one thing and just observe what was passing through, I began to relax and enjoy what I called "time out". I wasn't sure this qualified as meditation but I do know that I enjoyed my time outs and felt refreshed and renewed by them. Then the more I started taking time outs the fewer dogs went chasing through my mind and the quieter and deeper I could settle in to myself. I guess the point I want to make is meditation or quiet time or time out, shouldn't be work, it shouldn't be stressful, it should be whatever it is at that moment in time.

There are a few key elements to meditation or quiet time. The first is to be somewhere calm where you won't be disturbed. It may be your porch, your bedroom, your office with the telephone turned off, or for me outdoors among the trees or where I can hear water moving is my favorite. Close your eyes and take a couple of cleansing breaths. Follow the breath in to see where it is going or how shallow or deep it is. Then slowly let it out, again following it and observing how your body responds. Start at the top of your head and slowly moving down your body scan it to see where you are holding your tension. Common places are in the jaw or set of the teeth and the neck/shoulder area. If you find an area that is tight simply take your breath and your intention there and observe or give permission for your body to release the tension. When you have fully scanned your body and given it permission to relax start acknowledging the thoughts running through your mind and dismissing each of them as if they were the car you were chasing but knew you would never catch. Then imagine yourself resting in your peaceful place until the next car (thought) comes running through your mind. Eventually you will tire of chasing cars and be able to find a quieter, more subtle mind.

At this point you can end your meditation or if you want to go further you can ask your inner self a question? What do I need to feel more energy today? Who can help me get through this obstacle I've encountered? What do you, inner self, need from me today? What do we need to be healthier? Anything you are unsure of or any decision you are struggling with you can ask your inner self and receive direction or inspiration. However, if you decide to go to this level, which I would hope you will, be ready to trust the information you are given as a thought, a name, a phrase, a book you can read, however the information comes to you, act on it. That is how we build trust with our inner self. Each time that you receive a prompting from you inner self and you ignore it thinking "oh that person couldn't help", or "that doesn't make any sense", or "I don't want to bother them" you fail to recognize and acknowledge the authentic you. It is the authentic you that Craniosacral Therapy and Emotional Release Therapy are trying to help you uncover.

Stress

In 2005 the *Wall Street Journal* devoted an entire *Health Journal* section to an article entitled, "Secrets of Successful Aging". The article said, "Increasingly, researchers are viewing stress—how much stress we face in a lifetime, and how well we cope with it—as one of the most significant factors for predicting how well we age." The article went on to conclude that stress "kills" people as often, if not, more than smoking, drinking alcohol or not exercising. This is because stress is not just a mental emotional issue; it causes significant biological changes in the physical body.

A long-term study done at the University of London showed that chronic, unmanaged stress was six times more likely to cause cancer, and heart disease than smoking, high cholesterol and hypertension. In the magazine *Personality and Individual Differences* Vol. 9 a study done at the Mayo Clinic reported that for people with heart disease, psychological stress was the strongest predictor of future cardiac events. In other studies colleges have shown that in the weeks prior to and including final exams students tend to catch more colds and develop more infections than any other time of the semester. We can not separate the emotional state of the body from the physical state. The mind and the body are one entity and need to be treated as such.

Stress management courses have popped up in several different venues over the past few years. But I prefer the approach taught in the book, "One Minute Wellness" by Dr. Ben Lerner. "Stress management is an outside-in mechanical concept. The idea of managing stress is similar to the idea of managing or treating symptoms and illnesses. The outside-in, mechanical model treats unwanted health or disease with pills, surgery....to elevates the symptoms. Stress management involves treating stress with positive thinking or Prozac. So rather than calling it "stress management" we will call it *Peace Management*. Don't look to fight stress; instead build and manage peace so as to overcome and /or prevent stress."

Peace management starts with you taking responsibility for your emotions, your actions and your relationships. This is good news, by the way, because you can actually do something about *you*. You can't change others but you can change *you*. Again, this is what your craniosacral and emotional release therapies are helping you do.

Probably one of the greatest causes of stress is time or lack thereof. However, we all know we cannot create more time. Time management is another overwhelming topic that multiple companies have capitalized on to try to help people get organized, perform more optimally and enjoy life. At the very core of time management programs is purpose. If you don't know your purpose and what you are trying to accomplish you will waste valuable time trying to find something, but you aren't really sure what it is. Doing the craniosacral sessions, the writing assignments, and the mediation you will begin to have a sense of your authentic self and what it is you truly want out of this life. At that point you will need to focus on how you spend your time and what your distractions are pulling you away from that purpose.

One of the techniques I use with clients is for them to identify where they spend their greatest amount of time and then decide if that is an appropriate allotment of their time considering their purpose. Generally speaking the one thing that takes up a great deal of people's time is their career. With the technology of today people seem to always be plugged in and connected to work. Even if they happen to leave their work after an eight to ten hour day their smart phones are on while they are driving home so they can maximize that time returning telephone calls or responding to emails. Then at home finally they still can't bring themselves to turn the technology off. What if they miss a call or something unforeseen happens?

Once we have identified this over-expenditure of time in their life I ask them the question, "What is the worst thing that would happen if you were to adjust the amount of time you spend on "xyz" and only give it 50 hours a week instead of 75?" Normally at this point I will get considerable noise from the client while they try to justify why they have to spend the 75 hours. My job is to try to bring them into focus with what their self-created story is telling them versus what their real concern is. No matter what their response is I then ask, "And what is the worst thing that you can imagine would happen if indeed THAT happened?" This is a tedious process, but a highly effective one that helps us get to the bottom of why they have developed this compensation in their life that is distracting them from their authentic purpose.

Let's look back at Lisa in chapter 9. Once she was home and working on staying sober and changing her lifestyle things were going pretty good for her and her family, until the holidays. One evening I received a telephone call from Lisa. By the tone of her voice I could tell it wasn't a good evening. Her two teenage children both had friends over and were having a great time doing their thing. Wes was working late, even though he had promised to come home early so they could have a nice dinner together and then do some last minute Christmas shopping. They argued, Wes getting angry and frustrated, Lisa becoming angry and depressed. As Lisa told me the scenario of what was happening in her home, she added, "They really don't need me. I don't know why I'm trying so hard. They all have their own lives, except me."

I knew this was the old Lisa and her old story talking and helping her to understand that was not difficult, but I also knew this was a critical point in her wellness plan because the dynamics between Wes and her had obviously not changed even though she was changing in many ways. When Wes was gone for long hours or needed to work late after telling Lisa he would be home, Lisa interpreted this as "I'm not important", "no one loves me". She could change that interpretation, but it is also helpful to understand why Wes continued to repeat this scenario. *Key relationships in our lives can be a source of tremendous happiness, but they also can be the source of remarkable stress.*

After talking Lisa through her processing and interpretation of the situation and committing her to not go out for alcohol I placed a telephone call to Wes. After the usual pleasantries I explained to him that Lisa had called me and what we had discussed. I also told him I was concerned about her vulnerability. Wes immediately became defensive thinking that I was blaming him for the situation. Once I had let him

172

express his side of the story sharing his frustration of balancing work, family and Lisa's recovery process I asked if he would answer just one question for me and then I would let him get back to work. (He was struggling with the year-end finances of a large account that needed to be wrapped up before the holiday.) He told me he had time to answer one question.

So I asked, "What is the worst thing that would happen if you organized your desk, got up and walked out to your car and drove home right now?"

After a short course laugh he responded, "We'd probably lose this account."

Only having permission to ask one question, I asked, "And what is the worst thing that would happen if THAT happened?"

He sighed deeply and responded, "I don't know, but I don't want to find out either."

"Come on Wes you know what you tell yourself; just tell me, what is the worst thing that would happen if you lost the account?"

"I don't know, I guess maybe I would get fired." He paused, "But I don't even know that since I'm one of the principle partners. No, I think maybe what would happen is we would lose a lot of money and I would feel guilty and frustrated partly because I need the money to pay for all of Lisa's recovery bills."

"Okay, the firm would lose a lot of money and you would feel guilty and frustrated. In fact you may not be able to pay all Lisa's bills. So what is the absolute worst case scenario that would happen then?"

"Annette, stop it! Come on I have to get back to work." Wes was getting frustrated. This was good. It appeared he was getting frustrated with me, but I've been through this enough to know he was actually getting frustrated with coming to terms with his "story" and his authentic self. So I waited, not saying anything.

"Okay, worst case scenario, umm....I guess I would have to work harder to bring in another account that would make up the difference and that would be difficult and time consuming." He answered tersely.

"But it could be done?" I asked?

"Well yes, anything is possible." He half-barked in reply.

"So you could go home and enjoy your family and the holidays without the company falling apart or you losing your job?" I asked.

"Well, I suppose, but it is easier to just stay and get this done." He answered emphatically.

"Okay. One last question. You have indicated to me in the past that your top priorities in life are to be a good husband, an involved father and a good provider. Does that belief serve your priority's highest good? You don't need to answer that right now Wes. I'd just like you to think about it when you can. Thanks for your time and I hope you enjoy your holidays."

Two days later Wes called me to thank me for that conversation. He had decided to go home and enjoy his family. Why? Because I didn't try to force time management on him or try to make him feel guilty. But he went home because I helped him come to terms with an unrealistic story he was telling himself that did not serve his ultimate purpose of being a good husband and father as well as a good provider.

The next time you are feeling stressed out, try this little tool. Take a deep breath and ask yourself what is bothering you. Then ask the question, "What is the worst thing that could happen if "xyz" continues?" Then wait for the response. It might be immediate or it might take a few minutes. Then keep repeating the question until you feel like you have exhausted the issue and come to terms with the story you have created around your circumstances. Then ask one final question, "Does this thought serve my greater authentic purpose?"

By the time you finish this exercise you will have come to terms with yourself and will more clearly be able to define your next move which will empower you. Through this empowerment you will feel like you are back in the driver's seat of your life and your circumstances. That feeling alone will help you cope with the stress you are feeling.

Peace management is about managing moments that lead to your purpose. Learning to identify your purpose, manage the moment and how you think, feel and react to them is an inside out approach to life's stresses.

Chapter 13

A Few Final Words

I hope that through the words on these pages you have acquired a sense of my love and passion for craniosacral therapy and the somato emotional release work that goes along with it.

Sometimes when we have challenging things going wrong in our lives, rather it is physical or emotional, we look for the complicated answers because our pain seems complicated and disturbing to us. So when someone says why not try this or that, if it is not expensive, covered by insurance, well documented or performed by an expert, it is easy to push aside the suggestion.

It requires a certain amount of humility on our part to try something different or simple. Remember, to step away from the familiar to the possibilities the unfamiliar has to offer. The question I want to ask you is, "What do you have to lose by trying craniosacral therapy?" Perhaps you will lose a few of hours of your time, money; between $180-$300 for three sessions, or maybe, just maybe, a good deal of your pain and discouragement.

Since writing this manuscript I have had the opportunity to work with several patients experiencing cancer. I will not try and tell you CST will cure cancer...in fact, it will not. But it is a great adjunct therapy for detoxification of the brain from the chemotherapy, and it provides comfort and profound relaxation to the patient at a much needed time in their life. I've had the honor of helping a few patients pass on to the other side with less guilt or anxiety from processing past events in their life through somato emotional release. I cherish those experiences and may share them someday in another book. But, one thing that has been reinforced to me in my work with these cancer patients is that we **cannot** separate the physical and the emotional parts of our being. As I've mentioned earlier in this book, one affects the other and vice versa.

Thank you for taking the time to read this book. If I can be of further assistance in helping you to find answers in your search for wellness please contact me at awayoutofpain@gmail.com.

Printed in Great Britain
by Amazon

57302284R00106